The Acid Reflux Escape Plan

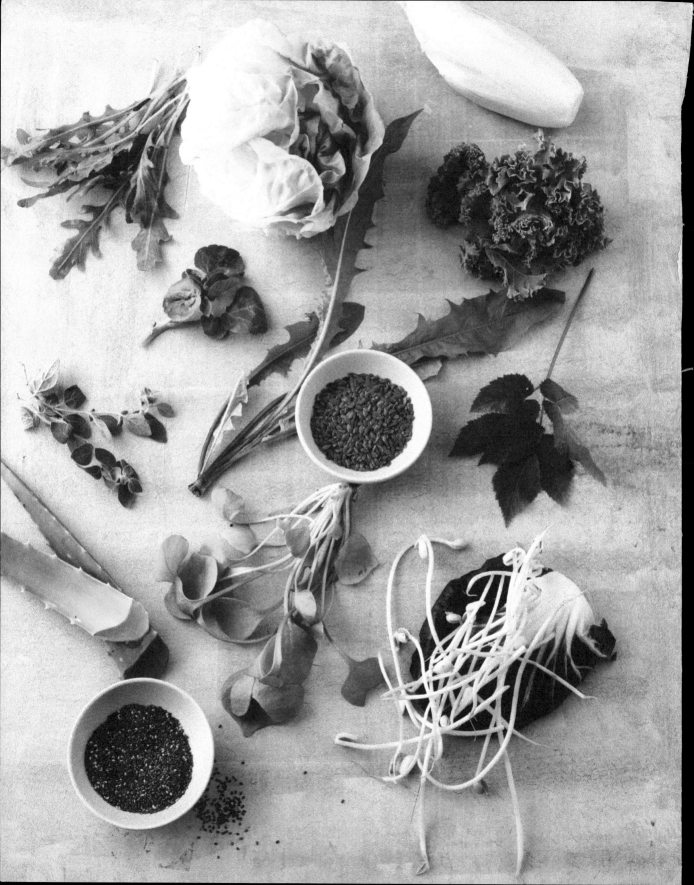

The ACID REFLUX escape plan

Two Weeks to Heartburn Relief

Karen Frazier

SONOMA PRESS

Photography © Stockfood/Jalag-Syndication/
Grossmann.Schuerle, cover and p.132; Stocksy/J.R.
Photography, p.2; Stockfood/Oliver Brachat,
p.8; Stocksy/Borislav Zhuykov, p.12; Stockfood/
Aran Goyoaga, p.14; Designua/Shutterstock, p.16;
Stockfood/Gräfe & Unzer Verlag/Eising Studio, p.26;
Stocksy/Laura Stolfi, p.42; Stockfood/Atelier Hämmerle,
p.60; Stockfood/ Gräfe & Unzer Verlag/Anke Schütz,
p.62; Stockfood/Valerie Janssen, p.66; Stockfood/
Olga Miltsova, p.73; Stockfood/ Gräfe & Unzer Verlag/
Joerg Lehmann, p.80; Stockfood/Victoria Harley, p.86;
Stockfood/ Gräfe & Unzer Verlag/Coco Lang, p.91;
Stockfood/Victoria Firmston, p.94; TK p.98; Stockfood/
People Pictures, p.98; Stocksy/ Davide Illini, p.105;
Stockfood/Gareth Morgans, p.110; Stockfood/Jalag-
Syndication/Janne Peters, p.116; Stockfood/Gareth
Morgans, p.123; Stockfood/Valeria Bismar, p.128;
Stocksy/Davide Illini, p.145; Stockfood/Mikkel Adsbol,
p.152; Stockfood/Andrew Young, p.160; Stockfood/
Gareth Morgans, p.168; Stockfood/Shaun Cato-
Symonds, p.175; Stockfood/Gräfe & Unzer Verlag/
Thorsten Suedfels, p.178; Stockfood/Magdalena
Hendey, p.182; Stockfood/Winfried Heinze, p.188;
Stockfood/Jo Kirchherr, p.193; Stockfood/Rua Castilho,
p.198; Stocksy/Rowena Naylor, p.202; Stockfood/Lars
Ranek, p.210; Stocksy/Laura Stolfi, p.216

ISBN Print 978-1-942411-15-4
eBook 978-1-942411-16-1

Contents

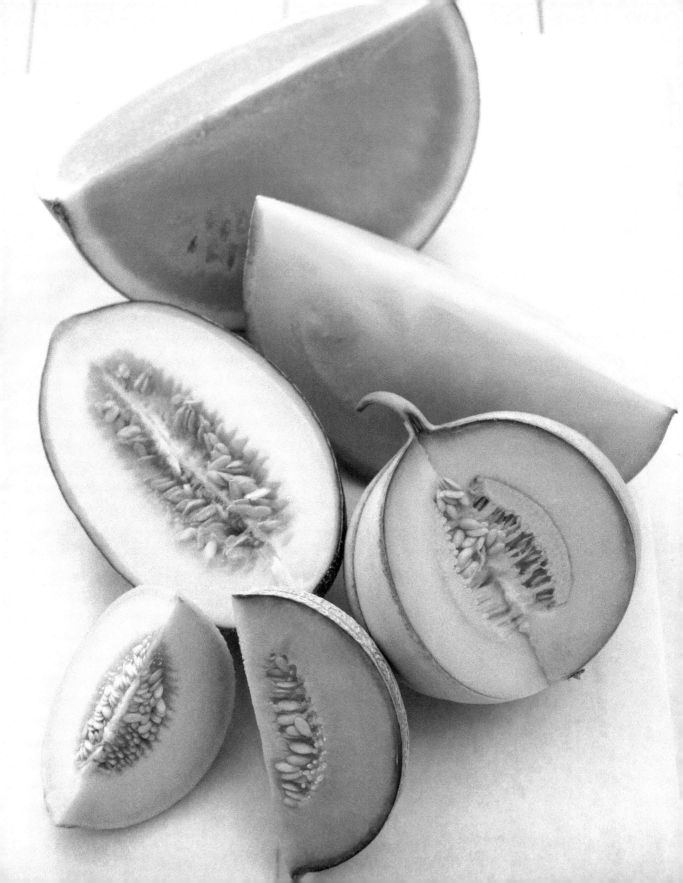

Introduction

Most people have experienced heartburn at some point in their lives. When that heartburn becomes a chronic, consistent problem, however, it can greatly affect your quality of life. Suddenly, every bite of food comes laden with the possibility of making you very uncomfortable, so you start to worry about everything you put in your mouth. That's no way to live.

If you are experiencing the symptoms of gastroesophageal reflux disease (GERD), you aren't alone. The National Institute of Diabetes and Digestive and Kidney Diseases notes that GERD affects about 20 percent of the population.

Along with causing discomfort during and after eating, GERD can affect other aspects of your life as well. For example, you may not sleep well if you experience symptoms during the night. And if left untreated, GERD can lead to serious health conditions, including esophageal cancer, respiratory problems, and other health issues.

With such a large swath of the population experiencing GERD, is it any wonder that grocery and drugstore shelves are stocked with over-the-counter treatments like proton pump inhibitors (PPIs), such as Prilosec and Prevacid, or histamine H_2 receptor antagonists (H_2 blockers), such as Tagamet, Pepcid, and Zantac? While these drugs may offer symptomatic relief of heartburn and GERD symptoms, they are not without risks and side effects themselves. In many cases, these drugs offer only short-term relief, leading to long-term use merely to control the symptoms.

According to an article in the medical journal *Therapeutic Advances in Gastroenterology*, while PPIs are the leading treatment for GERD, long-term use is not without risks, including rebound hypersecretion of acid. Likewise, the Mayo Clinic notes a long list of side effects associated with the use of H_2 blockers, such as blood vessel inflammation, joint pain, and difficulty breathing.

Clearly, controlling GERD symptoms with medications is not without risks. Therefore, before taking these medications, it is important to judge whether the risks outweigh the benefits.

What if there was a completely natural way to control your GERD and heartburn symptoms without exposing yourself to the risks inherent in taking medication? The good news is that there is a completely safe way to control your GERD symptoms, prevent diseases associated with long-term GERD flare-ups, and avoid taking risky medications. All you need to do is modify your diet.

Controlling your diet can help you completely control your GERD symptoms, leading you to feel so good that eating becomes a pleasure once again.

As you will discover in the following pages, what you eat strongly influences heartburn. Controlling your diet can help you completely control your GERD symptoms, leading you to feel so good that eating becomes a pleasure once again.

This cookbook and action plan are designed to help you discover and prepare the foods that will keep your symptoms at bay. It contains a meal plan designed to help you achieve symptomatic relief in just two weeks. The easy-to-follow recipes will provide you with delicious and easily prepared foods to help keep you feeling great for years to come.

If you've been suffering from frequent heartburn or any of the symptoms of GERD, then this action plan is for you. Following the plan and recipes will not only provide you with tasty meals, but it will also help you finally escape from acid reflux and all of the associated symptoms. That's because each of the recipes in this book avoids using ingredients that can cause heartburn, replacing them with delicious and healthy ingredients that nourish your body while helping you avoid pain.

For any food lifestyle change to be successful, it has to be sustainable. The recipes in this book are designed to offer you a long-term food plan that you can incorporate into your healthy lifestyle. Along with being flavorful, the recipes are quick, requiring less than 20 minutes of active time each. Likewise, the ingredients are simple and available in most grocery stores. The recipes don't call for any fancy or expensive ingredients, and you can prepare them in a kitchen stocked with basic equipment.

If you're ready to escape from the discomfort of acid reflux, then you've come to the right place. If you follow this plan, you will begin to experience symptom relief within two weeks. After the two-week period, you can customize the diet to eliminate your own personal triggers for a lifetime of heartburn relief without medication.

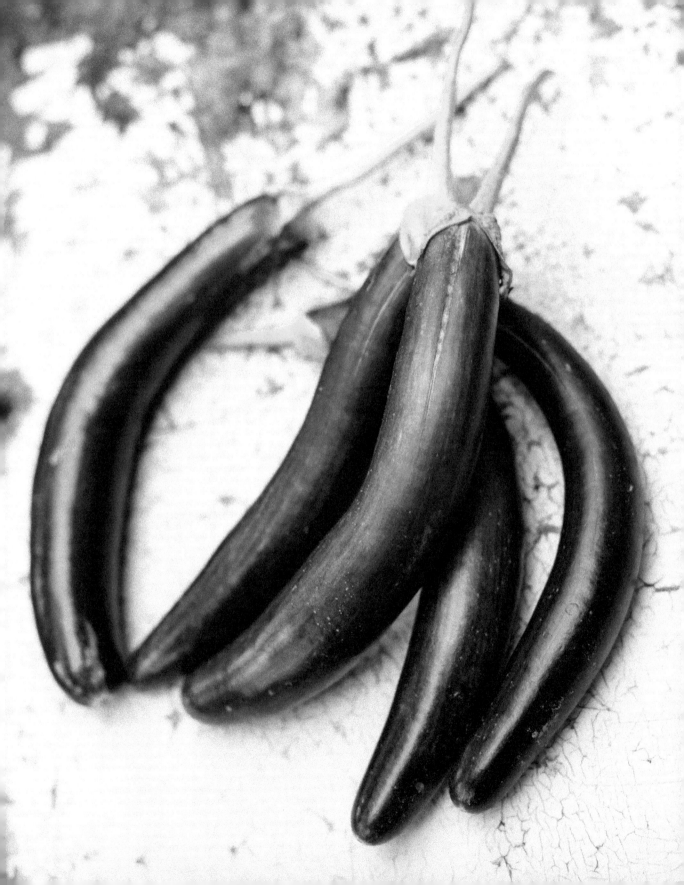

PART ONE

The Escape Plan

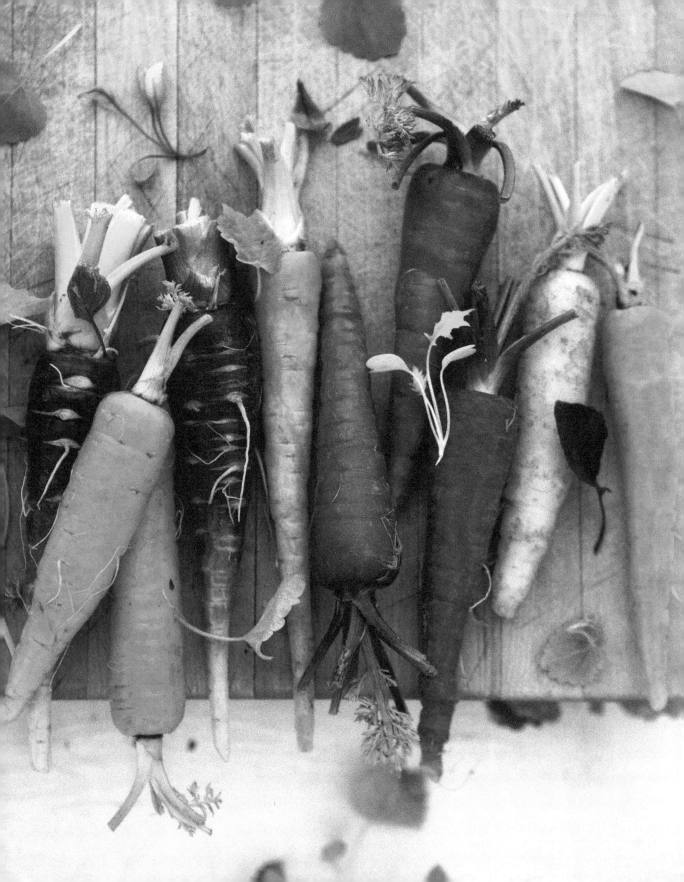

Chapter One

Understanding Acid Reflux and GERD

Reflux is a common health complaint, and it seems to be growing. A 2012 study conducted at the Norwegian University of Science and Technology noted about a 50 percent growth in GERD incidence in the 11-year span from 1995 to 2006.

With this upward trend in the prevalence of acid reflux, more and more people are experiencing the uncomfortable symptoms associated with the problem. For many, the problem is frequent, with symptoms recurring two times per week or more. Symptoms may be mild or severe.

A Widespread Problem

While the study cited previously was conducted as part of a greater Norwegian health study, the situation doesn't seem to be much different in the United States. According to Florida Hospital, about 40 percent of Americans report experiencing some type of acid reflux symptoms at least once a month, but what exactly is acid reflux?

Acid reflux is known by many names, including gastroesophageal reflux (GER), reflux, acid indigestion, acid regurgitation, and heartburn. According to the Cleveland Clinic, acid reflux occurs when stomach acid splashes up through the lower esophageal sphincter (LES), causing acid to enter the esophagus and contact its lining. This occurs because the LES, which functions as a valve that allows food to pass into the stomach but doesn't allow stomach contents to pass into the esophagus, fails to close properly. This allows for a backflow of stomach acid into the esophagus.

When food enters the stomach, it causes the stomach to secrete gastric acid, a combination of hydrochloric acid, sodium chloride, and potassium chloride. The acidic environment of the stomach is a very important factor in digestion, allowing your body to break down proteins for use in the cells.

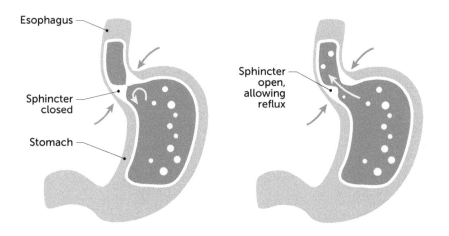

While the stomach is protected against its highly acidic environment, however, other organs and cell tissues are not. That's why, when stomach acid passes the wrong way through the LES, many people experience the symptoms of acid reflux.

If you experience acid reflux (GER) occasionally, it doesn't necessarily mean you have GERD. However, if the problem is persistent and frequent, occurring more than twice a week for a few weeks, then you may have GERD.

According to the National Institutes of Health, GERD may occur as the result of many factors, including:

- A weakened LES
- Increased abdominal pressure from obesity or pregnancy
- Certain medications including antihistamines, painkillers, sedatives, antidepressants, asthma medications, and calcium channel blockers
- Smoking
- Hiatal hernias

For this reason, certain populations may be more susceptible to experiencing GER or GERD, including:

- Infants
- Pregnant women
- People who are overweight or obese
- Smokers
- People who inhale secondhand smoke
- Older people
- People taking medications (see above)

Other factors may cause acid reflux symptoms as well, including:

- Spicy foods
- Acidic foods
- Alcoholic beverages
- Caffeinated beverages
- Carbonated beverages
- Foods that increase intra-abdominal pressure
- Foods that relax the LES
- Weight gain

Common Symptoms and Conditions

You are probably familiar with the most common symptoms of heartburn, such as chest and throat pain. However, there are also silent symptoms, and that means that many people with GERD may be unaware that they have the condition.

Symptoms

The National Institutes of Health and the Mayo Clinic note many symptoms of acid reflux and GERD, including the following:

PAINFUL BURNING. This is the most common and recognizable symptom of GERD. It typically occurs behind the breastbone and/or in the upper abdomen, and is caused by acid leaking through the LES.

BELCHING, NAUSEA, REGURGITATION, AND VOMITING. In some cases, the stomach acid leakage may be severe enough to trigger mild to severe nausea. In severe cases, vomiting may occur. The vomit may have streaks of blood in it. Likewise, acid may cause you to regurgitate small bits of food and acid, you may experience a painful burp that causes acid to enter your throat and mouth, or you may experience the taste of acid in the back of your throat and mouth.

BAD BREATH. As acid and food find their way out of the stomach and into the upper alimentary canal, they can cause foul-smelling breath.

DIFFICULTY SWALLOWING. The acid can also cause esophageal narrowing, scarring, or spasm, which may make it difficult to swallow.

SORE THROAT. Acid leaking into your throat may cause either painful burning in the throat or a persistent soreness. The acid may also affect your vocal cords, causing hoarseness, especially in the morning, or a dry cough.

DENTAL PROBLEMS. Acid working its way into your mouth may erode tooth enamel. You may also notice swelling, inflammation, or wearing of the gums.

Less Common Symptoms

The International Foundation for Functional Gastrointestinal Disorders (IFFGD) notes that people may experience less common or even silent symptoms, including:

- A sudden wash of saliva in the mouth, known as water brash
- The sensation of food sticking in the esophagus, known as dysphagia
- Frequent throat clearing
- Persistent cough
- Feeling like something is stuck in your throat

Conditions

A number of conditions may accompany GERD as well. These include the following.

LARYNGOPHARYNGEAL REFLUX (LPR)

The American Academy of Otolaryngology notes that in some cases, stomach contents may not only pass through the LES, but also through the upper esophageal sphincter, working their way into the throat and the nasal cavity. This causes a number of symptoms that many people don't typically associate with GERD, such as:

- Postnasal drip
- Frequent swallowing
- Sleep apnea
- Noisy breathing

In infants and children, LPR can also cause cyanosis (turning blue), spitting up, and breathing pauses. Some of these symptoms in very young children may be life threatening and require emergency care.

While LPR frequently accompanies GERD, it isn't present in every case of GERD. Likewise, people with LPR may or may not also have GERD. The two occur together commonly, but not exclusively.

RESPIRATORY PROBLEMS AND PULMONARY DISEASE

According to the *Physicians' Desk Reference,* a number of respiratory problems may occur in conjunction with GERD, including:

- Asthma and bronchospasm
- Persistent cough
- Sleep apnea

Likewise, an article in *Annals of Thoracic Medicine* notes that GERD can either trigger or exacerbate many pulmonary diseases, including:

- Ear, nose, and throat disorders
- Chest congestion
- Lung inflammation
- Bronchitis
- Pneumonia

These health issues may occur in conjunction with GERD because the stomach acid can enter the respiratory tract via LPR or aspiration, causing inflammation and damage to the tissues.

ESOPHAGITIS AND ESOPHAGEAL NARROWING

According to the Cleveland Clinic, repeated leaking of stomach acid into the esophagus can cause erosion or ulcers of the esophagus lining, known as esophagitis.

Over time, inflammation of the esophagus lining can lead to strictures, which are scarred patches that cause the passage to narrow.

BARRETT'S ESOPHAGUS AND ESOPHAGEAL CANCER

The Cleveland Clinic also notes that Barrett's esophagus is a complication associated with long-term GERD. Barrett's esophagus occurs when damage to the esophageal lining results in abnormal cellular changes. These changes can lead to the development of esophageal cancer.

ESOPHAGEAL CANCER

This may occur as a result of damage to cells from gastric acid, as well as from damage from smoking or heavy drinking. While esophageal cancer may initially be asymptomatic, as it progresses people may experience difficulty swallowing.

The Reflux Symptom Index

In *Dropping Acid: The Reflux Diet Cookbook & Cure*, Dr. Jamie Koufman and Dr. Jordan Stern developed the Reflux Symptom Index (RSI) as a tool that allows you to measure your GERD symptoms over the past month. It asks nine questions, allowing you to rank your symptoms on a scale of 0 to 5. On the following form, evaluate your own symptoms, circling the number that corresponds to the level of severity. Once you have done this, add up the total of the numbers you've circled. If your total is higher than 13, then you probably have GERD. Try following the two-week acid reflux escape plan outlined in this book, and then use the index to rate your symptoms again. Your total should be lower after you've eliminated the acid-causing foods. However, if it remains above a 13, you should seek medical consultation.

You can also use this index as you begin to determine your own personal GERD triggers. After testing a food for a few days, check your symptoms. If your number stays the same, that food probably isn't a trigger.

Within the last month, how did the following problem affect you?
(0–5 rating scale, where 0 = no problem and 5 = severe problem)

Hoarseness or problem with your voice	0	1	2	3	4	5
Clearing your throat	0	1	2	3	4	5
Excess throat mucus or postnasal drip	0	1	2	3	4	5
Difficulty swallowing foods, liquids, or pills	0	1	2	3	4	5
Cough after you ate or after lying down	0	1	2	3	4	5
Breathing difficulties or choking episodes	0	1	2	3	4	5
Troublesome or annoying cough	0	1	2	3	4	5
Sensations or something sticking in your throat	0	1	2	3	4	5
Heart burn, chest pain, indigestion, or stomach acid coming up	0	1	2	3	4	5

Total

From *Dropping Acid: The Reflux Diet Cookbook & Cure*, reprinted by permission of Dr. Jamie Koufman and Dr. Jordan Stern.

WHEN SHOULD I SEE A DOCTOR?

With so many over-the-counter cures for heartburn and GERD, many people choose to self-treat when symptoms flare up. In the case of very occasional bouts of indigestion (less than once a month), this approach may work as long as you are using only an antacid, like Tums or Rolaids. However, if you have a condition that is severe enough to warrant the use of stronger medications, like H_2 blockers and PPIs, then you may want to think twice before self-treating.

While these medications are available over the counter, they may have associated side effects. Furthermore, certain medications may interact with other medications that you are taking. Therefore, it is important that your doctor has all of the necessary information about all of your health conditions and treatments.

If you experience any of the following warning signs, seek medical care:

- **Chest pain:** While chest pain may indicate GERD in some cases, it also may be a sign of a more serious problem, such as a blockage in the blood vessels of the heart or even a heart attack. Always seek immediate medical attention if you experience chest pains, especially if they are accompanied by other symptoms such as shortness of breath, arm pain, and jaw pain.

- **Recurring symptoms:** If you experience recurrent bouts of heartburn, you may have GERD as opposed to simple gastroesophageal reflux.

- **Symptoms unaffected or minimally affected by antacids:** See a doctor if your antacids stop providing relief.

- **Persistent throat or respiratory symptoms:** If you have a cough, sore throat, hoarseness, or other symptoms that affect you for more than a week, see your doctor.

- **Symptoms of increasing severity:** Visit your doctor if your symptoms continue to increase in severity.

- **Keep a journal of your symptoms,** including details on when they occur, how long they last, and how severe they are. This information is important for your doctor to make an accurate diagnosis, since GERD symptoms can often mimic other conditions such as sinusitis or allergies. To confirm his or her diagnosis, your doctor may perform tests, such as inserting a small nasal tube to measure acid over 24 hours, a digestive system X-ray, or an endoscopy. These tests can help your doctor assess your condition and prescribe appropriate treatments.

Popular Medical Treatments

While this book is about diet and lifestyle management to minimize or eliminate reflux symptoms, some people may still benefit from medical management of their condition. Work in conjunction with your doctor to find the least invasive, most effective form of management possible to supplement this dietary lifestyle. Explain to your doctor that you are trying to manage your GERD through diet alone, and ask for two weeks to try out a diet before adding medical treatments. Then, discuss all of the available options with your doctor in order to reach the treatment that works best for you. The goal is to minimize medical intervention as much as possible in order to naturally treat your symptoms.

Medications

Currently, the most commonly used treatment for acid reflux and GERD is the prescription of medications.

ANTACIDS

Many doctors prescribe over-the-counter antacids, such as Maalox, Tums, or Rolaids. These antacids contain simple agents that neutralize excess stomach acid. The National Library of Medicine notes that antacids are effective for occasional bouts of heartburn that occur after you eat. For some people, the body adapts to antacids, and they eventually need to take more and more to have the same effect. As your body adapts to the neutralizing effect of the antacids, it begins to produce more acid in response, leading to the need for more antacids. This develops into a loop of dependency, and before they know it, many people are quickly going through large containers of antacids.

Antacids are not without side effects. Depending on the antacid you take, you may experience diarrhea or constipation. Taking large amounts of antacids may lead to kidney stones or loss of bone mineralization. They may also interact with certain medications.

H₂ BLOCKERS

These medications, which include Zantac, Tagamet, Axid, and Pepcid, work by blocking how much acid the stomach produces. Typically, you need to take these medications 30 to 90 minutes before eating, but the drug may help symptoms for as long as 24 hours. The medications may cause side effects, such as headaches, diarrhea, dizziness, and rash. The drugs in this class may also interact with other medications. Lower-dose H₂ blockers are available over the counter.

PPIS

Proton pump inhibitors reduce the amount of acid your stomach produces. Medications in this class include Prilosec, Nexium, Prevacid, and several others. Generally, you take one tablet in the morning, about 30 minutes before you eat. You need to take PPIs daily, sometimes for as long as eight weeks (or, in some cases, even longer). PPIs allow time for the esophagus to heal from damage caused by acid.

PPIs may cause side effects, especially with long-term use. These side effects may include tendency toward fractures, infection, nausea, constipation, and itching. They may also interact with other medications. PPIs are available in lower doses over the counter.

Quitting PPIs can cause rebound hyperacidity, where you experience even more severe symptoms than you did before you started the PPIs. This is usually temporary, but is an unpleasant side effect of the medication.

BACLOFEN

Your doctor may prescribe Baclofen, which strengthens the LES. It is usually prescribed in conjunction with other types of medications, such as PPIs, in cases of severe GERD. It has many side effects, including drowsiness, dizziness, weakness, and difficulty breathing. It is available by prescription only, and may interact with other medications you take.

SURGERY

In severe cases, your doctor may recommend surgical intervention, such as using a surgical device to tighten or strengthen the LES. These surgeries are performed laparoscopically, leaving a small incision site and decreasing post-operative recovery time. However, they still have the same types of risks as other surgeries requiring general anesthesia. The

Society of American Gastrointestinal and Endoscopic Surgeons notes that anti-reflux surgery, while highly effective, may not be appropriate for every patient.

According to the Cleveland Clinic, for patients with hiatal hernias complicating their GERD, surgery on the hernia may be indicated. This is the case only if the hernia is strangulated, or if it is contributing so significantly to GERD that the disease cannot be medically managed in any other fashion.

LIFESTYLE CHANGES

Your doctor may also recommend making lifestyle changes, including altering your diet, losing weight, eating smaller meals, and elevating the head of your bed. These lifestyle changes will be discussed in Chapter Two.

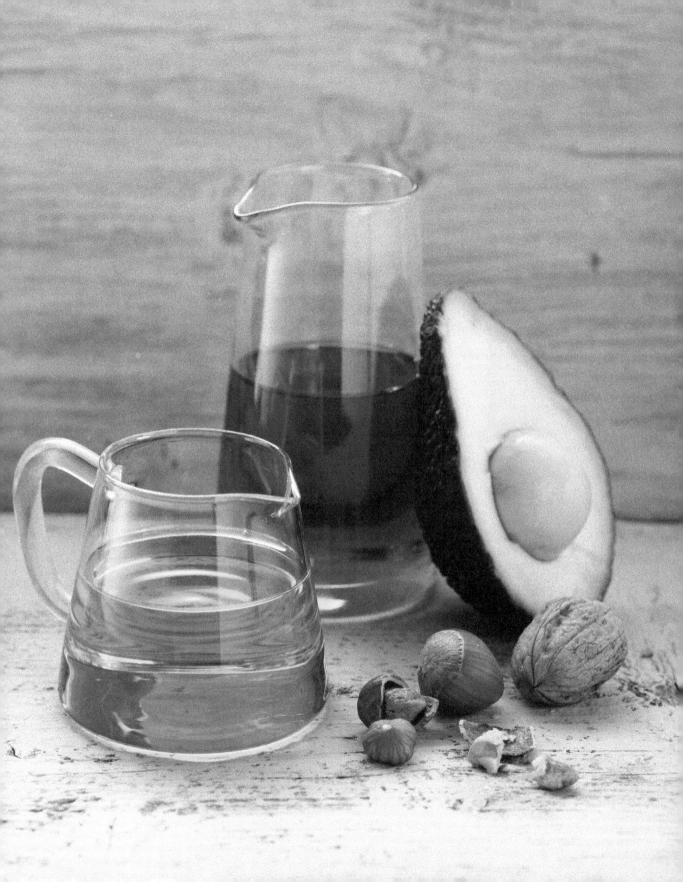

Empowered Eating and Healthy Living

If you've been struggling with symptoms of acid reflux, then chances are you know just how problematic they can be. While medical management and certain medications can help temporarily, many people experience escalating symptoms and issues in spite of the medications they take. More symptoms trigger a need for more medication, which triggers more symptoms in a spiral of pain and medication.

Are you ready to stop the madness? By making some simple dietary and lifestyle changes, you can break this cycle and gain control of your GERD symptoms once and for all.

Neutralizing Acid Reflux
with Smart Eating

The way you eat can have a significant effect on your acid reflux symptoms. Changing your eating habits and selecting the right foods make a big difference. The McKinley Health Center at the University of Illinois at Urbana-Champaign lists a number of lifestyle changes you can make to help manage your acid reflux.

EAT SMALLER MEALS. Eating large meals causes increased abdominal pressure, which can force acid past the LES and into your esophagus, leading to symptoms of GERD. Instead, eat five to six small meals and snacks per day. This ensures you get all of the nutrients your body needs without creating the abdominal pressure that can trigger reflux.

LIMIT FAT. Fried foods are one of the biggest triggers of acid reflux because of their fat content. Fat in the diet relaxes the LES, allowing gastric acid to seep into the esophagus. Fat also slows how quickly the stomach empties after eating it, which can increase abdominal pressure. A low-fat diet is very helpful in reducing symptoms of GERD.

AVOID ACIDIC FOODS. While this will be discussed in depth later, it bears mentioning now as well. Highly acidic foods, such as citrus fruits and juices, tomatoes, and vinegars, can all increase stomach acid, which can increase acid reflux.

MAKE WATER YOUR DRINK. Carbonated beverages, caffeinated drinks, coffee, tea, and alcohol can all cause acid reflux. For example, carbonated beverages increase abdominal pressure, which may force acid through the LES. Alcohol, caffeine, coffee (even decaf), and tea all weaken the LES. Drinking water at the end of each meal can help dilute any stomach acid.

WATCH THE SPICES. Spicy foods, such as chiles, onions, garlic, hot mustard, mint, and horseradish are all well-known acid reflux triggers. This is likely because the spices irritate the esophageal lining.

CUT OUT THE CHOCOLATE AND THE MINT. If you're a lover of Thin Mint cookies, then Girl Scout cookie-selling season could be causing your GERD. Both chocolate and mint weaken the LES muscle.

MAINTAIN YOUR GUT BIOME. In *Fast Tract Digestion: Heartburn*, Norman Robillard, PhD, studies the relationship between intestinal flora and heartburn. Dr. Robillard argues that small intestinal bacterial overgrowth (SIBO) caused by consumption of foods that ferment in the gut can cause gas buildup, which exerts pressure on the LES, leading to GERD. Because of this, maintaining healthy bacteria in the gut is essential. Eat foods that contribute to healthy gut bacteria, such as low-fat plain yogurt or kefir.

CONSIDER ELIMINATING FODMAPS. A 2010 study in the *World Journal of Gastroenterology* concluded that GERD and irritable bowel syndrome (IBS) may have a common or overlapping cause. One diet that has worked very well for people with IBS is a low-FODMAP diet, as reducing FOD-MAPs in the diet also reduces symptoms of IBS, according to a study that appeared in the medical journal *Gastroenterology* in January 2014. FODMAP is an acronym for groups of simple carbohydrates called "fermentable oligosaccharides, disaccharides, monosaccharides, and polyols." These short-chain carbohydrates attract water when they sit in the gut, and they produce a lot of gas as they ferment. A low-FODMAP diet removes the source of gas that can increase abdominal pressure, triggering symptoms of acid reflux. While FODMAPs are beyond the scope of this book, you can read about them in *The Low-FODMAP 28-Day Plan* by Rockridge Press.

LOWER YOUR CALORIES. If you are overweight, then this can contribute to heartburn flare-ups. Being obese, particularly around your mid-section, increases abdominal pressure, which may lead to heartburn.

DON'T EAT LESS THAN THREE HOURS BEFORE BEDTIME. Lying down after eating relaxes the LES and allows stomach acid to flow upward, so if you have acid reflux, going to bed shortly after eating can be a big trigger. Instead, make sure you end your last meal at least three hours before you go to bed and/or lie down in order to keep the stomach contents where they belong: in your stomach.

BAKE, BROIL, GRILL, OR STEAM YOUR FOODS. Cooking meats and vegetables using these methods lowers the fat in the foods, which helps keep GERD in check.

The Relationship Between Food pH and Acid Reflux

In *Dropping Acid: The Reflux Diet Cookbook & Cure*, Dr. Jamie Koufman and Dr. Jordan Stern make the case that the pH of foods eaten has a direct correlation to the triggering of reflux symptoms. According to the authors, acidic foods (those with a lower pH) are more likely to trigger reflux, while those foods with a higher pH will not.

pH measures acidity or alkalinity in substances, including food. The pH scale runs from 0 to 14. Substances with a neutral pH (such as water) have a pH of 7. Battery acid, an extremely acidic substance, has a pH of 0. Liquid drain cleaner, which is so alkaline it is caustic, has a pH of 14.

Naturally, you won't be eating battery acid or liquid drain cleaner. However, foods also fall toward the middle of the spectrum, ranging from a pH of about 2 for citrus juices and vinegar, to a pH of about 8 for baking soda and eggs. Drs. Koufman and Stern note that foods with a pH of about 4 or less are likely triggers of acid reflux, so it is important to avoid foods that fall below that pH on the scale. However, for people with severe GERD, you may need to avoid foods that have a pH that falls below 5 (see Appendix A: The FDA's Food pH List).

Food Allergies, Sensitivities, and Intolerances

People who consume foods to which they are allergic, intolerant, or sensitive may trigger GERD symptoms merely by ingesting that food. For example, people with an intolerance to gluten or wheat, such as celiac disease, often report experiencing GERD symptoms, which go away once they eliminate gluten from their diet.

Dr. Stephen Wangen, Director of the IBS Treatment Center, notes that food allergies are one of the most frequently overlooked causes of reflux. He notes that the top food allergies that may trigger reflux include dairy, eggs, soy, and gluten.

For this reason, it is important to avoid any foods to which you are allergic, sensitive, or intolerant. All of the recipes in this book can be adjusted for people with intolerances. For example, if you are allergic to dairy, replace milk with nonfat rice milk and eliminate cheese.

COPING WITH CRAVINGS: HELP!

Whenever you alter your diet, chances are some cravings will arise. In some cases (such as caffeine, alcohol, or cigarettes), those cravings come from an actual physical addiction. In others, the craving may be more emotional or mental.

Coping with Cravings Arising from Physical Addictions

▸ **Follow a plan.** If you're quitting smoking, then you may wish to work with your doctor for a medically managed plan, such as nicotine patches. Avoid nicotine gum that is mint flavored, because mint may cause heartburn.

▸ **Taper off slowly.** If you're quitting coffee or some other caffeinated beverage (such as energy drinks, cola, or tea), your best bet is to withdraw slowly before you start this food plan. Taper your consumption, first by mixing your coffee half and half with a decaffeinated coffee, and over the course of two or three weeks tapering off until you're not drinking it at all. Once the physical addiction to the caffeine in coffee has been surmounted, you can then deal with the cravings for the flavor of coffee, tea, or cola with some of the tips listed to the right.

▸ **Ask your doctor for help.** If you are quitting alcohol and you believe you have a drinking problem, medical management is important. Talk to your doctor to develop a strategy so you don't experience severe withdrawal symptoms.

Coping with Emotional/ Mental Cravings

▸ **Wait it out.** Often, a craving will go away if you just ignore it. Give it 30 minutes and see if it goes away. If it doesn't, then look for a similar food to satisfy your craving. For example, if you're craving pickles, it's probably the vinegar you want. Instead, have a small salad with about a tablespoon of vinaigrette to give you the flavor without all of the acid.

▸ **Visualize or meditate.** As soon as a craving hits, picture yourself doing something you really love. Stay with the visualization until the craving goes away. Alternatively, meditate.

▸ **Engage in doing something you love.** Of course, you don't have to visualize if you're in a position to get up and do something. Listen to music. Dance. Hang out with your kids. Find an activity that takes your mind away from your craving and immerse yourself in it.

▸ **Smell something pleasant that doesn't smell like food.** A 2012 study in the medical journal *Appetite* showed that people with chocolate cravings noted a significant reduction in the craving when sniffing jasmine.

FOODS TO ENJOY AND AVOID

Food or Food Group	Noteworthy Information
Alcoholic beverages	Relaxes LES
Margarine, shortening	Too high in fat
Caffeine	Stimulant
Carbonated beverages	Acidic, increases abdominal pressure
Chocolate	Stimulant, causes reflux
Citrus fruits and juices	Acidic
Chiles, peppers, and hot sauce	Known to trigger reflux
Cream sauces	Too high in fat
Dairy	Avoid high-fat dairy, such as butter, cheese, whole milk, full-fat yogurt or sour cream, and cream. Some recipes may contain very small amounts for flavor.
Herbal or regular tea	Known to trigger reflux
Fried foods	Single largest trigger of reflux and heartburn
Fruit	All except those listed below
Garlic	Known reflux trigger
Meat, beef	Avoid fatty cuts higher than 15% fat
Meat, pork	High in fat
Mint	Known reflux trigger
Onions	Known reflux trigger
Peppers, green	Known reflux trigger
Spicy foods	Known reflux trigger

ABSOLUTELY AVOID

FOODS TO ENJOY AND AVOID

Food or Food Group	Noteworthy Information
Apples, green	Acidic, causing problems in some people. Eat red apples instead.
Artificial sweeteners	Limit to 1 to 2 teaspoons per day.
Bell peppers, red	Less than ¼ pepper per day
Butter	Limit to less than 2 tablespoons per day.
Cheese, Parmesan or sharp cheddar only	Limit to 2 tablespoons per day or less. Use primarily as a flavoring.
Chamomile tea	One cup per day or less
Coffee, decaffeinated	One cup per day or less
Cucumber	May trigger reflux in some people.
Mustard, Dijon	Less than 1 tablespoon per day for flavoring
Pepper, black	May trigger reflux in some people. Use only in very small amounts—one shake of the pepper shaker.
Raisins	Don't eat by themselves. Eat only in conjunction with whole grains, which will absorb some of the acid. Limit to less than 2 tablespoons per day.
Sesame seeds	1 tablespoon per day or less to add flavor
Tomatoes	May trigger reflux in some people. May use a small amount for flavoring, but eat in conjunction with starchy foods to blunt the effect. Less than 2 tablespoons of tomato sauce per day.
Vinaigrette	1 tablespoon per day or less

CONSUME WITH CAUTION

FOODS TO ENJOY AND AVOID

Food or Food Group	Noteworthy Information
Agave nectar	Low-glycemic sweetener, adds flavor
Avocado	Excellent source of fiber and vitamins; great stand-in for high-fat dairy in salad dressing
Apples, red	Fuji, Red Delicious, four per week or fewer
Bananas	A very small number of people may be sensitive, so if it seems to be a trigger for you, omit it.
Beef, extra-lean cuts	Less than 15% fat
Breads and muffins	Non-fruit versions only
Celery	Helps control appetite
Cereal	Whole-grain
Citrus zest	Citrus flavor without the acid
Corn	All kinds, including cornmeal
Eggs, large	Four per day or fewer
Fennel	Improves stomach/digestive function
Fish and shellfish	Baked, broiled, steamed, or grilled but not fried
Fish sauce	Adds flavor
Ginger	Fresh or powdered
Grains, whole	Absorb acid
Herbs and spices	All but peppers, chiles, and mint
Honey	Good for soothing heartburn
Legumes	Chickpeas, beans, pinto beans, black beans, etc.
Maple syrup	Adds flavor
Melon	Cantaloupe, honeydew, or watermelon
Milk	Nonfat, 1%, 2%, or soy

FOODS TO ENJOY AND AVOID

Food or Food Group	Noteworthy Information
Miso	Adds flavor
Mushrooms	All varieties
Oatmeal	Absorbs acidity
Olive oil	1 to 2 tablespoons daily
Olives	Low acid
Pasta	With low-acid sauce
Pears	Ripe only, four or fewer per week
Popcorn	Air-popped only, no butter
Poultry	Skinless only, not fried
Poultry broth or stock	Homemade is best
Rice	All types, although brown rice is best
Salt	This is not a low-sodium diet. However, if you have a history of hypertension, you may need to lower the salt in recipes.
Soy sauce	Great way to add flavor
Sugar	Moderate amounts of brown and white sugar add flavor.
Tofu	An excellent protein source for vegetarian meals
Vegetables, cruciferous	Cabbage, broccoli, cauliflower, broccoli rabe, broccolini
Vegetables, green	All, except for cucumbers and green peppers
Vegetables, other	Any unless otherwise noted
Vegetables, root	Potatoes, rutabaga, carrots, turnips, etc. Noted exception: no onions
Yogurt	Low-fat, plain

Lifestyle Changes to Escape Heartburn

Diet is only part of the picture in eliminating acid reflux. You can make a number of lifestyle changes to help minimize or eliminate your symptoms.

MANAGE YOUR STRESS. A 2004 study in the journal *Psychosomatic Medicine* concluded that life stresses increase the incidence and severity of GERD flare-ups. Therefore, stress management is essential in managing your condition. There are numerous ways you can manage your stress, including meditation, doing breathing exercises, stretching, or engaging in yoga. If you choose yoga for stress management, make sure you do it either before you eat or more than three hours after eating so inverted postures don't trigger a flare-up of GERD, which would defeat the purpose of the yoga.

SIT AND STAND UP STRAIGHT. Your mother always told you to stand up straight, but she probably didn't realize she was teaching you a life strategy for managing GERD. Having an upright posture supports the LES and keeps the stomach contents where they belong. Slouching increases abdominal pressure, encouraging gastric acid to head toward the LES, which is exactly where you don't want it.

RAISE THE HEAD OF YOUR BED. One of the reasons acid reflux occurs so often when you're sleeping is because when you're lying down, the gastric juices are free to wander away from your stomach. If your LES is relaxed, they just may make their way into your esophagus. Propping the head of your bed up slightly by putting supports under the legs, or by sleeping with pillows propping you up from your chest upward, can help relieve those nighttime bouts of acid reflux.

DON'T WEAR TIGHT CLOTHES. Tight clothing, especially clothes that are tight around the middle, increases abdominal pressure, forcing the gastric juices upward to press on the LES. Choose looser-fitting clothes that don't pull around the middle.

EXERCISE. Working out helps relieve stress, which is a factor in GERD. Likewise, it can help you lose weight if you are overweight, which is also a cause of acid reflux.

QUIT SMOKING. Smoking is a big trigger of acid reflux because it weakens the LES and increases stomach acid. This double whammy is one of the worst things you can do to exacerbate your GERD, so quitting can definitely improve it. Talk to your doctor about strategies for quitting.

SLOW DOWN AND ENJOY YOUR MEAL. Eating quickly may trigger GERD as well. That's because when you eat quickly, you increase your abdominal pressure quickly. Instead, practice mindful eating, paying attention to every bite and putting your fork down between bites.

KEEP A LOG. Track the foods you eat and the symptoms you experience. Then, look in your journal for patterns. If you notice a specific food that you eat before a bout of GERD, chances are it's a personal trigger for you and you should probably eliminate it from your diet.

DISCUSS YOUR MEDICATIONS AND SUPPLEMENTS WITH YOUR DOCTOR. Some medications and supplements—including over-the-counter remedies—may trigger GERD. Talk to your doctor about the medications you are taking and look for options that won't trigger your condition.

REMAIN UPRIGHT AFTER EATING. When you look at the mechanics of acid reflux, it's easy to understand why lying down or reclining might send stomach contents upward towards the esophagus. Try to sit up straight or stand up for a few hours after eating to ensure the food stays where it belongs. However, don't run right out for a jog, because exercising right after eating may also cause reflux. Walking is fine.

GET PLENTY OF SLEEP. Sleep deprivation is hard on your body in a number of ways, including increasing stress. As previously mentioned, stress contributes significantly to reflux. Try to get at least seven to eight hours of sleep per night.

DO SOMETHING YOU LOVE. Along the lines of stress management, taking time to find ways to really engage in things you enjoy is the best remedy for stress. Find something you love to do and make time to do it several times a week.

Defensive Dining: Eating Out with GERD

RESTAURANT FOOD CAN BE SO TEMPTING. It smells good and looks even better. Every time the server walks by with a plate of food, you can feel yourself salivating. Unfortunately, if you're not careful, giving in to those temptations can leave you with a severe flare-up of heartburn.

PLAN AHEAD. When you go to a restaurant, check out the menu and find items that fit your needs. Call ahead to restaurants and explain you have a special diet. Ask if you can order items off the menu.

DON'T GO WHEN IT'S BUSY. If possible, visit the restaurant during off hours when it isn't busy. That way, you can chat with the waiter, and the kitchen may have time to prepare a special order.

ORDER WITHOUT SAUCE. Order meals without sauce or butter. Good menu items include things like steamed or grilled fish or poultry, steamed vegetables without seasoning, and plain rice or potatoes. Emphasize that the only seasonings you can have are salt and herbs. If you have a salad, instead of ordering a dressing, ask for oil and vinegar and mix them yourself at the table so you can go light on the vinegar.

TAKE SOMETHING TO SHARE. If you're going to an office party or a friend's house, offer to bring something to share. Then, make a food you can eat and take it with you. Make plenty so others can have it.

TALK TO THE HOST. If you feel comfortable, let the host know your dietary restrictions. Most people hosting friends in their home want to be gracious and provide foods others can eat. Think of it this way: If you were vegetarian, you wouldn't hesitate to share your dietary restrictions with a host or hostess. This is the same idea.

MEDICATE STRATEGICALLY. While this book is about helping you manage your symptoms with diet, it's understandable that you will sometimes give in to temptation. If you're going to your favorite restaurant to have your favorite food and you know you're going to give in, then consider taking an H_2 blocker 30 to 90 minutes before you go.

Holiday Help

Often the holidays, with their big meals and fast-paced life, can aggravate GERD. Fortunately, you can navigate the holidays with minimal flare-ups using the following strategies.

YOU BE THE HOST. One of the least stressful (from a food perspective) ways to ensure you eat the way you want to during the holidays is to host meals yourself. To save yourself some stress, instead of cooking the whole meal, you can cook a few dishes that you can eat, and then ask friends and family to bring their favorites.

TAKE FOOD TO PARTIES. When you go to parties, bring something to share or discreetly bring a few snacks of your own and munch on them. Bring some celery sticks, a hard-boiled egg, or some carrots. People won't notice that you're not eating from the party buffet.

TAKE TIME TO RELAX. The holidays are stressful, and stress can cause a flare-up of acid reflux. During the holiday hustle and bustle, be sure to take time for yourself. Spend 20 minutes soaking in the bathtub or curl up for a half hour with a favorite book. Be sure to take a little bit of time for yourself every day, no matter what you've got going on.

STAY HYDRATED. Keep a bottle of water with you at all times. That way, when others are sipping on some holiday cheer, you have something to drink as well. Plus, drinking water will help dilute stomach acid and keep your energy up.

BE CHOOSY AT THE BUFFET. Most buffets have a few good choices, such as turkey, salads, or vegetables. Fill your plate with foods that won't cause a flare-up of your symptoms. Be sure to remove the skin on poultry, and keep lean beef to small amounts. Don't fill up too much, either. Try to continue eating several small meals throughout the day, which will make you less hungry when you get to a big meal.

PACE YOURSELF. This recommendation goes for both food and activities. The food was covered above, but be sure you pace yourself with activities as well. There's no need to say yes to every event or invitation. Allow yourself time to slow down as much as you need and enjoy the holiday season.

TIPS AND TRICKS FOR IMMEDIATE HEARTBURN RELIEF

If you're in the midst of an attack, all you want is for the heartburn to go away. Here are some strategies to help immediately.

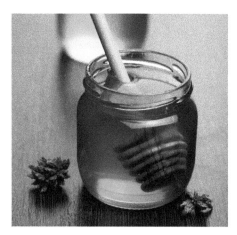

▶ **Take a tablespoon of raw honey.** Raw honey is anti-inflammatory and can help soothe the esophageal lining when acid splashes it.

▶ **Take an antacid.** There's no mystery about this one—millions of people take antacids on a daily basis. While the antacid may help cool your heartburn right away, long-term use can actually exacerbate symptoms, so it's best to reserve this intervention for the worst flare-ups.

▶ **Take 1 teaspoon of baking soda in 1 cup of water.** Baking soda is highly alkaline, and it will neutralize the acid when your GERD flares up. It works in a manner similar to antacids, so once again you want to keep this to a minimum so you don't ultimately create more stomach acidity with long-term use.

▶ **Chew sugar-free gum.** Be sure you choose a non-mint gum, since mint exacerbates GERD. This simple act can help get saliva flowing, reducing stomach acidity.

▶ **Drink aloe juice.** You can find aloe at the health food store. It is soothing and calming, and should soothe GERD. Be warned, however, that it is also a laxative.

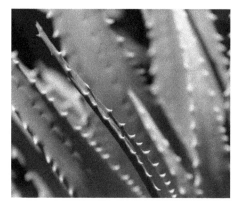

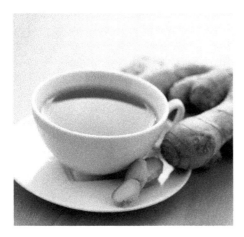

▶ **Chew some deglycyrrhizinated licorice (DGL).** You can find DGL tablets at the health food store. While the results of studies about DGL for heartburn are mixed, a great deal of anecdotal evidence exists suggesting it soothes heartburn.

▶ **Have a teaspoon of yellow mustard.** Although it contains a little bit of vinegar, mustard itself is alkalizing, and neutralizes the acid. If you can't swallow a teaspoon of mustard by itself, mix it with some water. And don't use spicy mustard or hot mustard, because the heat may worsen the GERD.

▶ **Drink ginger tea.** Ginger is great for the stomach, calming a number of stomach ailments, from nausea to acid reflux. Grate some fresh ginger and simmer it in water for 30 minutes. Strain, and drink the tea.

▶ **Drink chamomile tea.** Chamomile tea can help calm and soothe inflammation associated with acid reflux. However, in some people it is a reflux trigger, so if you are one of those people, avoid it.

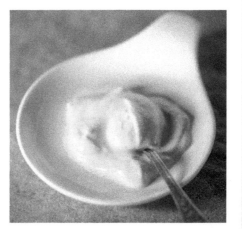

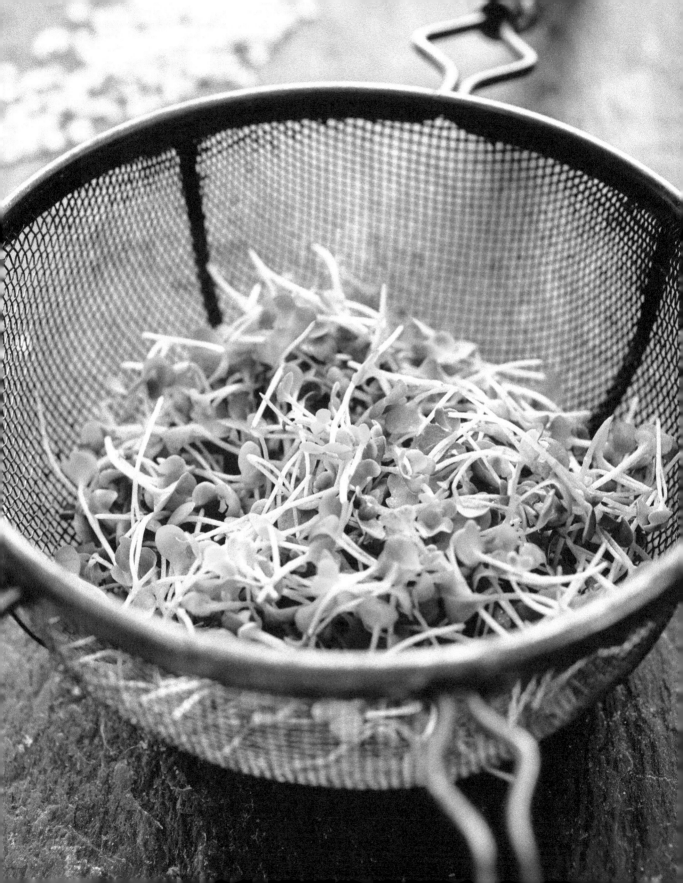

Chapter Three

The Acid Reflux Escape Plan

This chapter contains two weeks' worth of menus that will empower you to take control of your acid reflux symptoms. Acid reflux is a stressful condition, because you never know when something you eat will trigger extreme discomfort and burning pain. However, the meal plan will help you kick-start your new way of eating, allowing you to lead a more normal, stress-free life. Because you'll learn exactly what to eat, eating will no longer be a stressful venture that can lead to pain. Instead, eating once again becomes a pleasurable and flavorful activity.

Making the Acid Reflux Escape Plan Work for You

This meal plan is your ticket to escaping acid reflux. By combining the elements of choosing foods that don't aggravate reflux and managing abdominal pressure with smaller portions, you will soon be free of burning pain after you eat.

- ▶ The acid reflux meal plan allows for five small meals per day, including a small breakfast, a mid-morning snack, a small lunch, a mid-afternoon snack, and a small dinner. Eating five times per day will keep you from growing hungry in spite of the small portions, and the meals will satisfy all of your body's nutritional needs.
- ▶ The meal plan uses leftovers as much as possible in order to minimize meal preparation. In some cases, dinner leftovers may be tomorrow's lunch.
- ▶ The recipes rely on inexpensive and easy-to-find ingredients so people on fixed budgets can afford the plan.
- ▶ Most of the meals require less than 30 minutes of active time, although some may spend a bit longer than that in the oven or on the stovetop. For those with a slightly longer cooking time, however, they still don't require you to do any more work. Because they are so quick and easy, even the busiest professionals and parents will have time to prepare healthy, acid-reducing meals.
- ▶ The recipes are very easy to follow, and they don't require any complicated techniques or special equipment.

Setting Yourself Up for Success

If you're ready to take control of your acid reflux and get started with the plan, there are several steps you can take to set yourself up for success.

ELICIT THE SUPPORT OF FRIENDS AND FAMILY. Let your friends and family know about the changes you are about to make in your lifestyle and eating. Explain to them exactly why you are doing this, and ask that they support you. This is especially important if your family will be eating the same meals you do every evening. Ask your family, friends, or significant other to provide support as you go about the acid reflux plan. Having a supportive group of family and friends will help motivate you to continue.

COMMIT TO CHANGE. While the initial stage of the Acid Reflux Escape Plan is a two-week eating plan, in order to manage symptoms for life, you need to commit to a lifestyle change. Thinking about eating a certain way long-term and never being able to have some of your favorite foods again on a regular basis may seem overwhelming. However, as you begin to feel better and experience fewer symptoms, you will feel more motivated to continue.

The best way to commit to making the changes necessary for lifetime management of acid reflux is by realizing you aren't on a temporary diet—you are changing your lifestyle in order to have a less stressful, pain-free life.

STOCK THE PANTRY. One of the best ways to stay on track is to stock your pantry, refrigerator, and cupboards with healthy, low-acid foods. Keep tempting foods out of the house so you don't succumb to cravings. If you do keep acid-producing foods in the house for others, isolate them in a cupboard you never enter so that you don't have to see them on a daily basis.

ADAPT YOUR OWN RECIPES. While the recipes in this cookbook are a great start at an acid-free lifestyle, eventually you'll want some more variety. Once you have the basic principles of an acid-free lifestyle, you can begin to adapt some of your favorite recipes to meet your needs.

MAKE MEALS AHEAD. The Acid Reflux Escape Plan requires that you prepare homemade meals every day for yourself. However, everyone has experienced just not wanting to cook once in a while. To save yourself from heading out for a fast-food burger with ketchup, tomatoes, onions, and grease, stock your freezer with a few low-acid meals that you've made ahead of time. Then, all you need to do is thaw and reheat, and you'll have a quick and easy low-acid meal.

COOK ONCE, EAT TWICE (OR MORE). To save yourself from having to cook daily, employ the cook-once-eat-twice method. Make a meal (double the recipe if you have to), and then refrigerate the leftovers for tomorrow. For recipes that freeze well, you can freeze any leftovers for those nights you don't want to cook.

STICK TO RECOMMENDED PORTIONS. Since overeating can lead to increased abdominal pressure, having small portions is a key part of this plan. The portion sizes of the recipes in this book have been designed to provide small yet satisfying meals that won't increase abdominal pressure significantly.

TRACK YOUR SYMPTOMS. Sometimes when symptoms disappear, it's difficult to recall that you ever had them in the first place. That's why keeping track of symptoms can be very helpful for staying on track. If you can look back and recall the symptoms you once had, you will see what the diet is doing for you, which can help you stick to your guns when you get a craving.

REEVALUATE PERSONAL HABITS. Whether you smoke, you're a habitual coffee or soda drinker, you're overweight, or you enjoy a gin and tonic every night before bed, it's important to realize that many of these habits can lead to increased acid reflux symptoms. While diet is one part of the equation, managing lifestyle choices is an equally important aspect. Therefore, it's important to find ways to manage these habits in order to fully manage the symptoms of GERD. If necessary, work with your doctor to help change the habits that are contributing to your symptoms.

Two-Week Meal Plan

The meal plans outlined below make liberal use of leftovers. If you also serve these meals to your family, double a recipe in order to have the leftovers. All dinners either have a main dish and a side dish, or a main dish and a dessert. If the main dish doesn't have vegetables, then it has a simple vegetable side dish. Otherwise, it has a dessert. Dessert isn't available for every meal due to the necessity of keeping meals small. Recipes included in this book are indicated with an asterisk (*).

WEEK 1

MONDAY

Breakfast: Melon Smoothie*

Snack 1: 6 baby carrots with Creamy Ranch Dressing*

Lunch: Savory Turkey Burgers*

Snack 2: Baked Sweet Potato Chips*

Dinner: Red Beans and Rice*; ½ cup steamed broccoli

TUESDAY

Breakfast: Maple-Spice Oatmeal*

Snack 1: Apples with Honey-Yogurt Dip*

Lunch: leftover Red Beans and Rice

Snack 2: Baked Sweet Potato Chips*

Dinner: Ground Turkey, Mushroom, and Fennel Soup*; 1 scoop low-fat vanilla ice cream

WEDNESDAY

Breakfast: Canadian Bacon Breakfast Sandwich*

Snack 1: slices from ½ zucchini with Creamy Ranch Dressing*

Lunch: leftover Ground Turkey, Mushroom, and Fennel Soup

Snack 2: Apples with Honey-Yogurt Dip*

Dinner: Baked Cod with Ginger-Melon Salsa*; Honey-Roasted Asparagus*

THURSDAY

Breakfast: Zucchini and Mushroom Omelet*

Snack 1: Sweet and Spicy Popcorn*

Lunch: leftover Baked Cod with Ginger-Melon Salsa

Snack 2: celery sticks (from 1 stalk) with Creamy Ranch Dressing*

Dinner: Asparagus, Spinach, and Chicken Roulade*; Coffee Granita*

FRIDAY

Breakfast: Melon Smoothie*

Snack 1: 6 baby carrots with Spinach Dip*

Lunch: leftover Asparagus, Spinach, and Chicken Roulade

Snack 2: Sweet and Spicy Popcorn*

Dinner: Mushroom and Fennel Stew over Egg Noodles*; Coffee Granita*

SATURDAY

Breakfast: French Toast*

Snack 1: 1 cup honeydew melon balls

Lunch: leftover Mushroom and Fennel Stew over Egg Noodles

Snack 2: celery sticks (from 1 stalk) with Spinach Dip*

Dinner: Baked Halibut with Sour Cream-Dill Topping*; Creamed Spinach*

SUNDAY

Breakfast: Banana Crêpes*

Snack 1: Zucchini and Smoked Salmon Rounds*

Lunch: New England Clam Chowder*

Snack 2: hardboiled egg

Dinner: Southwestern Shrimp, Mushrooms, and Rice*; iceberg lettuce with Creamy Ranch Dressing*

WEEK 2

MONDAY

Breakfast: Maple-Spice Oatmeal*

Snack 1: hardboiled egg

Lunch: leftover New England Clam Chowder

Snack 2: Zucchini and Smoked Salmon Rounds*

Dinner: Hamburger Stroganoff*; Honey-Roasted Asparagus*; Maple-Ginger Pudding*

TUESDAY

Breakfast: Melon Smoothie*

Snack 1: banana

Lunch: Spaghetti with Ground Turkey and Broccolini*

Snack 2: 6 baby carrots with Orange-Honey-Dijon Dressing*

Dinner: Pork Tenderloin with Apples and Fennel*; leftover Maple-Ginger Pudding

WEDNESDAY

Breakfast: Canadian Bacon Breakfast Sandwich*

Snack 1: celery sticks (from 1 stalk) with leftover Orange-Honey-Dijon Dressing

Lunch: leftover Hamburger Stroganoff

Snack 2: Baked Sweet Potato Chips*

Dinner: Creamy Asparagus Soup*; Gingered Baked Pears*

THURSDAY

Breakfast: Maple-Spice Oatmeal*

Snack 1: Baked Sweet Potato Chips*

Lunch: leftover Creamy Asparagus Soup

Snack 2: ½ red apple and ½ cup low-fat cottage cheese

Dinner: Ginger-Glazed Scallops with Sugar Snap Peas*; leftover Gingered Baked Pears

FRIDAY

Breakfast: Pumpkin Pancakes*

Snack 1: Shrimp Salad on Melba Toast*

Lunch: leftover Pork Tenderloin with Apples and Fennel

Snack 2: banana

Dinner: Maple-Soy Glazed Salmon*; roasted asparagus

SATURDAY

Breakfast: Zucchini and Mushroom Omelet*

Snack 1: ½ cup nonfat plain yogurt with ½ cup honeydew melon balls

Lunch: leftover Maple-Soy Glazed Salmon; roasted asparagus

Snack 2: leftover Shrimp Salad on Melba Toast

Dinner: Baked Chicken Tenders*; 6 baby carrots with leftover Orange-Honey-Dijon Dressing

SUNDAY

Breakfast: French Toast*

Snack 1: ½ red apple; ½ cup low-fat cottage cheese

Lunch: Ginger Chicken and Rice Soup*

Snack 2: slices from ½ zucchini with leftover Orange-Honey-Dijon Dressing

Dinner: Turkey Breast Cutlets with Mashed Potatoes and Mushroom Gravy*; Baked Butternut Squash*

Most of the foods in the meal plan feature recipes included in this book. Some very simple foods, such as hardboiled eggs, cottage cheese, and steamed broccoli aren't included as recipes in the book.

Shopping List: Week 1

PRODUCE

- Apples, Fuji (2)
- Arugula (2 ounces)
- Asparagus (1½ pounds)
- Avocado (1)
- Bananas (2)
- Broccoli (1 bunch)
- Carrots, baby (8-ounce bag)
- Carrots, large (9)
- Celery (9 stalks)
- Cilantro, fresh (1 bunch)
- Dill, fresh (1 bunch)
- Fennel (4 bulbs)
- Ginger (1 knob)
- Lemons (6)
- Lettuce, iceberg (1 head)
- Lime (3)
- Melon, honeydew (1)
- Mushrooms, button (1½ pounds)
- Mushrooms, cremini (10 ounces)
- Mushrooms, shiitake (1 pound)
- Oranges (3)
- Parsley, fresh (1 bunch)
- Potato, russet (1)
- Potatoes, sweet (2)
- Rosemary, fresh (1 bunch)
- Spinach, baby (10 ounces)
- Spinach (22 ounces)
- Tarragon, fresh (1 bunch)
- Thyme, fresh (1 bunch)
- Zucchini (2)

PANTRY ITEMS

- Allspice, ground
- Bay leaves
- Cinnamon, ground
- Cloves, ground
- Coriander, ground
- Cornstarch
- Cumin, ground
- Dill, dried
- Fish sauce
- Flour, all-purpose
- Ginger, ground
- Honey
- Maple syrup, pure
- Mustard, Dijon
- Nonstick cooking spray
- Noodles, egg
- Nutmeg, ground
- Oats, rolled
- Olive oil, extra-virgin
- Popcorn, air-popped
- Rice, brown
- Salt
- Sesame oil, toasted
- Soy sauce
- Sugar, brown
- Thyme, dried
- Vanilla, alcohol-free

DAIRY AND EGGS

- Eggs, large (1 dozen)
- Milk, nonfat (½ gallon)
- Sour cream, nonfat (20 ounces)
- Yogurt, nonfat plain (24 ounces)
- Yogurt, Greek, nonfat, plain (20 ounces)

CANNED/JARRED/BOXED

- Chickpeas (14-ounce can)
- Clam juice (8-ounce bottle)
- Kidney beans (14-ounce can)

FROZEN

- Corn (16-ounce package)
- Ice cream, nonfat vanilla (1 pint)
- Peas (16-ounce package)
- Spinach (16-ounce package)

MEAT/POULTRY/FISH

- Bacon, Canadian (1 slice)
- Chicken breast, boneless, skinless (1 pound)
- Chicken wings (3 pounds)
- Clams (18-ounce can)
- Cod (four 4-ounce fillets)
- Halibut (1 pound)
- Salmon, smoked (6 ounces)
- Shrimp, medium (1 pound)
- Turkey bacon (2 ounces)
- Turkey breast, cutlets (1 pound)
- Turkey breast, ground (1½ pounds)

OTHER

- Bread, whole-wheat (1 loaf)
- Buns, hamburger, whole-wheat (4)
- Coffee, decaffeinated (brewed, 2 cups)
- English muffins, whole-wheat (1 package)
- Rice, brown (cooked, 2 cups)

Shopping List: Week 2

PRODUCE

- Apples, Fuji (3)
- Asparagus (4 pounds)
- Bananas (2)
- Broccolini (8 ounces)
- Carrots, baby (8-ounce bag)
- Carrots, large (4)
- Celery (6 stalks)
- Cilantro, fresh (1 bunch)
- Fennel (1 bulb)
- Ginger (1 knob)
- Lemon (1)
- Lime (1)
- Melon, honeydew (1)
- Mushrooms, cremini (22 ounces)
- Oranges (2)
- Parsley, fresh (1 bunch)
- Peas, sugar snap (2 cups)
- Pears (2)

- Potatoes, russet (2)
- Potatoes, sweet (2)
- Rosemary, fresh (1 bunch)
- Squash, butternut (1)
- Tarragon, fresh (1 bunch)
- Thyme, fresh (1 bunch)
- Zucchini (2)

PANTRY ITEMS

- Baking Powder
- Bread crumbs, panko
- Noodles, egg
- Rice, brown
- Rosemary, dried
- Sage, dried
- Spaghetti
- Tarragon, dried

DAIRY AND EGGS

- Buttermilk, nonfat (1 pint)
- Cottage cheese, low-fat (8 ounces)
- Eggs, large (1 dozen)
- Milk, nonfat (1 gallon)
- Sour cream, nonfat (8 ounces)
- Yogurt, nonfat, plain (6 ounces)
- Yogurt, Greek, nonfat, plain (12 ounces)

CANNED/JARRED/BOXED

- Pumpkin purée (14-ounce can)

FROZEN

- Peas (16-ounce package)

MEAT/POULTRY/FISH

- Bacon, Canadian (1 slice)
- Beef, ground, extra-lean (1 pound)
- Chicken, breast, boneless, skinless (1½ pounds)
- Chicken wings (3 pounds)
- Pork, tenderloin (1 pound)
- Salmon (four 4-ounce fillets)
- Salmon, smoked (6 ounces)
- Scallops (1 pound)
- Shrimp, baby, cooked (8 ounces)
- Turkey breast, cutlets (1 pound)
- Turkey breast, ground (½ pound)

OTHER

- Melba toast
- Rice, brown, cooked (2 cups)

Reintroducing Foods

Not all foods are heartburn triggers for all people. While the initial two weeks of this plan (and most of the recipes in this cookbook) eliminate all triggers, there are some foods that, while triggers for other people, may not necessarily be triggers for you.

Once you've gone through the initial two weeks, you can begin to reintroduce certain foods into your diet to see if they are triggers for you. These are the foods that are on the Consume with Caution list, such as red peppers and small amounts of hard cheeses.

After the two weeks, try reintroducing one food at a time to see how it affects you. Eat a small portion of the food at one meal and then track your symptoms for three or four days. If you have no symptoms, you can try having a little more and tracking your symptoms for a few more days. If you continue to have no symptoms, you can assume this is a food that is safe for you to eat in limited amounts.

Use the chart on the next page to identify your own personal triggers.

IDENTIFYING PERSONAL TRIGGERS

Food	pH Level	Quantity Consumed	Physical Reactions
Canned tomatoes	4.1 – 4.6	¼ cup	Woke up with hoarse voice

Kitchen Equipment

While the recipes in this cookbook require very little special equipment, some items will help you have more success and make cooking easier.

BAKING PANS. You'll need at least two large nonstick baking sheets. You'll also need baking pans in three different sizes: 9-inch loaf pan, 9-inch square pan, and 9-by-13-inch pan.

BLENDER. You'll need a countertop blender for smoothies, sauces, and puréeing soups. Any blender will do. Try to find one with multiple speeds.

CAST IRON SKILLET. Cast iron skillets are extremely affordable. They also go from the stovetop to the oven without pause, and when properly seasoned, they have a perfect nonstick surface. You'll need at least a 12-inch skillet. You can use other sizes as well.

DUTCH OVEN/STOCKPOT. Choose a large pot that will hold lots of liquid to make soups and stews. Try to find one that doesn't have plastic handles so you can transfer it to the oven from the stovetop. Enameled cast iron or cast iron work well for this purpose.

PARCHMENT. Parchment paper, which you can find in the grocery store in the aisle with the plastic wrap, is a great way to line baking sheets to make them nonstick.

SAUCEPANS. You'll need small, medium, and large saucepans.

UTENSILS. You'll need sharp knives, peelers, cutting boards, measuring cups and spoons, wooden spoons, spatulas, and other cooking utensils as well.

Pantry Items

Having a well-stocked pantry allows you to be able to quickly pull together meals. Removing items that tempt you will help keep you on track. The following items are essential components of a well-stocked anti-acid pantry.

HERBS AND SPICES

- Allspice, ground
- Cinnamon, ground
- Cloves, ground
- Coriander, ground
- Cumin, ground
- Ginger, ground
- Italian seasoning, dried
- Lemon zest, dried (if you can find it)
- Nutmeg, ground
- Orange zest, dried (if you can find it)
- Oregano, dried
- Rosemary, dried
- Sage, dried
- Salt
- Tarragon, dried
- Thyme, dried

CONDIMENTS AND OIL

- Fish sauce
- Mustard, Dijon
- Olive oil, extra-virgin
- Nonstick cooking spray
- Sesame oil, toasted
- Soy sauce

GRAINS AND LEGUMES

- Bread, English muffins, and hamburger buns, all whole-wheat
- Crackers, low-fat
- Flour, gluten-free (if gluten sensitive)
- Flour, all-purpose white or wheat
- Melba toast
- Noodles, egg
- Pasta (spaghetti, linguine)
- Popcorn kernels
- Rice (brown, white, basmati)

BAKING STAPLES

- Baking soda
- Baking powder
- Honey
- Maple syrup, pure
- Sugar, brown
- Sugar, granulated
- Sugar, powdered

GERD-FRIENDLY PANTRY SUBSTITUTIONS

Remove	Replace With
Garlic powder/garlic salt	Basil, cumin, Dijon mustard, Italian seasoning
Lemon or lime juice	Lemon or lime zest
Chili powder	Cumin, coriander
Paprika	Cumin
Cayenne	Cumin
Shortening/butter	Extra-virgin olive oil, nonstick cooking spray
Ketchup	Anchovy fillets or anchovy paste, Creamy Ranch Dressing (page 190), Dijon mustard, fish sauce, soy sauce, toasted sesame oil
MSG	Salt, soy sauce, fish sauce
Mayonnaise	Nonfat Greek yogurt, Low-Fat Mayonnaise Replacement (page 196)
Onion powder	Ginger, salt, cumin, coriander
Salad dressing	Salad dressing made with nonfat plain yogurt, low-fat milk, and herbs, Ginger-Lime Vinaigrette (page 186)
Canned tomatoes	Dijon mustard, soy sauce, fish sauce, anchovy paste
Pepper	Oregano, Italian seasoning, cumin, thyme
Oil-packed tuna	Water-packed tuna
Chicken broth (made with onions)	Homemade Chicken Broth (page 185) or Vegetable Broth (page 184)
Barbecue sauce	Liquid smoke, fish sauce, soy sauce, Dijon mustard

Cooking Advice for Acid Reflux Sufferers

After the initial two-week meal plan, chances are you will want to branch out to other foods and meals. The following cooking advice will help you keep your meals low-acid.

Use Fat Sparingly

Fatty foods are known acid reflux triggers. Therefore, when you cook it is essential that you use fat sparingly. You don't need to make your meals fat free, but try to keep your meals to less than 2 tablespoons of fat.

TO REDUCE FAT:
- Choose lean cuts of meat.
- Always trim visible fat from meats.
- When cooking high-fat ground meat, brown the meat in a skillet, then drain in a colander and rinse to remove any excess fat.
- Use just 1 or 2 tablespoons of oil when sautéing meat and vegetables.
- Eliminate sources of fat such as mayonnaise or whole milk.
- Limit cheese to 2 tablespoons or less per serving.
- Choose low-fat dairy products instead of full-fat.

Mix Acidic Foods with Alkaline Foods

If you took high school chemistry, then you may remember the part about mixing acids with bases to neutralize the acidic properties of the acid and the caustic properties of the bases. This is the same principle behind antacids. However, you can also do this with food. For example, if you have some vinaigrette, be sure you put high-pH foods such as asparagus, chickpeas, or kale on your salad. If you have raisins in your oatmeal, neutralize them with a little bit of nonfat milk. Mix a small amount of tomatoes with a small amount of cheese to minimize the acid.

Serve Water with Meals

Drinking water while you eat dilutes the gastric juices that result from the foods. Watering down these gastric juices can help prevent the burn from entering your esophagus.

Use Cooking Methods That Trim the Fat

Broiling, baking, roasting, grilling, and steaming are all methods that don't require you to add extra fat. You can sauté with a little bit of oil, but skip frying and deep-frying. You can minimize the amount of fat during sautéing by using nonstick pans and nonstick cooking spray.

Use Flavorings That Don't Trigger GERD

While garlic, onions, peppers, vinegar, citrus juice, and tomatoes can all trigger GERD, there are a number flavorings and methods you can use that add tremendous flavor without the acid. Try the following:

- ▸ Dry mustard
- ▸ Soy sauce
- ▸ Fish sauce
- ▸ Grated Parmesan cheese
- ▸ Sesame seeds
- ▸ Brown sugar
- ▸ Pure maple syrup
- ▸ Molasses
- ▸ Citrus zest
- ▸ Dried herbs and spices
- ▸ Fresh herbs and spices
- ▸ Dried mushrooms
- ▸ Chicken broth
- ▸ Vegetable broth
- ▸ Roasting meats and vegetables to develop deep flavor
- ▸ Deglazing a sauté pan by pouring a little liquid into the hot pan and scraping the browned bits from the bottom of the pan
- ▸ Allowing vegetables and meats to caramelize in the pan, turning a deep golden brown

Make Your Own Broth

Commercial chicken, beef, and vegetable broths are all made with onions, garlic, and black pepper. Cooking your own and freezing it in single-use containers eliminates the acid-causing ingredients that are a problem in GERD. See the recipes for Chicken Broth (page 185) and Vegetable Broth (page 184).

Learn Helpful Substitutions

Learn which flavors and substances can be substituted to eliminate GERD-causing ingredients and fats. For example, replace oil with apple-sauce in baking recipes and use nonfat yogurt in place of butter or cream in cream sauces.

Adapt Your Own Recipes

As you go along, you'll discover ways to adapt your own recipes so they taste just as good as they always did, but don't cause GERD.

Freeze Leftovers

To minimize the amount of cooking you have to do, refrigerate or freeze leftovers so you will always have meals at the ready. You can also use leftovers for next-day lunches or snacks.

Measure Portions

When you do store leftovers, measure them into individually sized portions so you aren't tempted to overeat. Since overeating can trigger heartburn, it's essential that you stick to small portion sizes.

Plan Simple Snacks

Snacks don't need to be difficult. They can be as simple as salted popcorn, a banana, some oatmeal, or a few carrot sticks.

Always Shop with a List

Shopping with a list will keep you from getting distracted by all the tasty-looking foods at the grocery store and keep you on track for your eating plan.

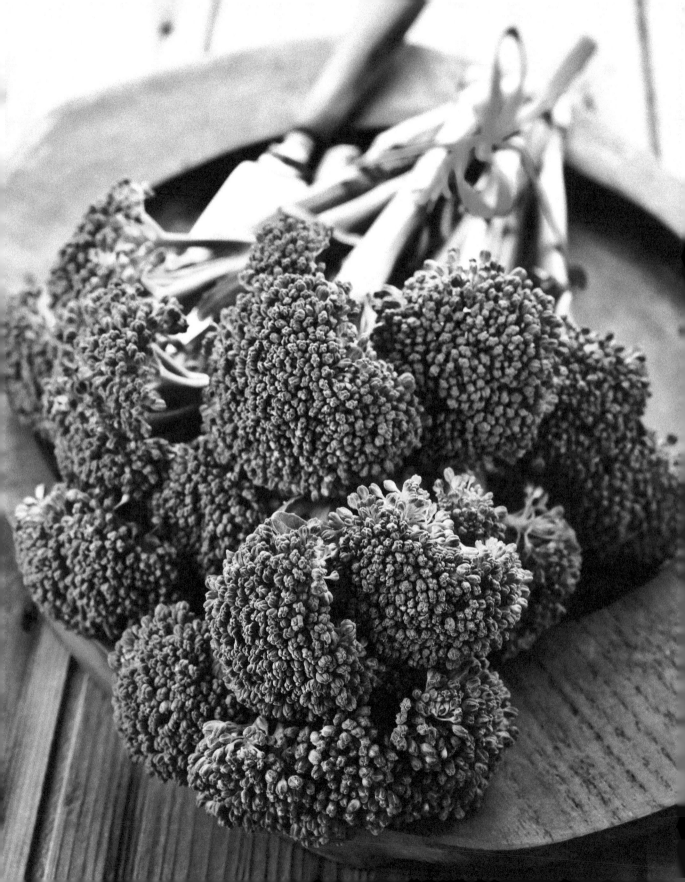

PART TWO

The Recipes

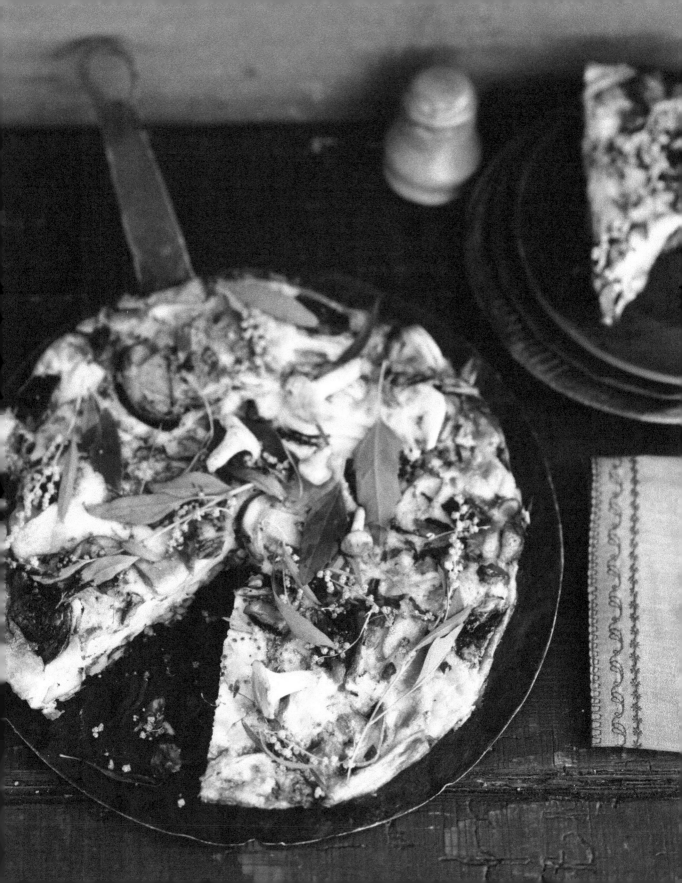

Breakfast and Brunch

Melon Smoothie

PREP TIME: 5 MINUTES / COOK TIME: 0

Mixing up a smoothie is a great way to start the day. It takes less than five minutes to make, so it gets you out the door quickly in the morning. It also has healthy protein to sustain your energy until your midmorning snack. Serves 2

⅛ honeydew melon, peeled and chopped

1 cup nonfat milk

¼ cup plain nonfat yogurt

2 tablespoons honey

Combine all the ingredients in a blender and process until smooth, about 1 minute. Serve.

SUBSTITUTION TIP: *If you're allergic to dairy, you can replace the milk with rice milk and the yogurt with silken tofu. The shake will taste great, but it won't aggravate your allergies.*

PER SERVING Calories: 269; Total Fat: 1g; Saturated Fat. 1g; Sodium: 180mg; Carbohydrates: 53g; Fiber: 0g; Protein: 12g

Maple-Spice Oatmeal

PREP TIME: 5 MINUTES / COOK TIME: 5 MINUTES

If it's a hot breakfast you're craving, then oatmeal is a fantastic way to start the day. This lightly spiced oatmeal is sweet from the cinnamon and a hint of maple syrup. The oats have plenty of fiber, giving them staying power to keep you satisfied throughout the morning. Serves 2

1 cup rolled oats

¾ cup water

¾ cup nonfat milk

Pinch salt

½ teaspoon ground cinnamon

1 tablespoon pure maple syrup

1   In a medium saucepan, bring the oats, water, milk, and salt to a rolling boil over high heat.

2   Reduce the heat to medium. Cook, stirring occasionally, for 5 minutes.

3   Remove the pan from the heat and stir in the cinnamon and maple syrup. Let the oatmeal stand for 2 minutes before serving.

SUBSTITUTION TIP: *If you like raisins in your oatmeal, you can add 2 table-spoons when you add the syrup and cinnamon. However, don't do this during the initial two weeks, and make sure raisins aren't a personal acid reflux trigger.*

PER SERVING Calories: 216; Total Fat: 3g; Saturated Fat: 0g; Sodium: 132mg; Carbohydrates: 40g; Fiber: 4g; Protein: 8g

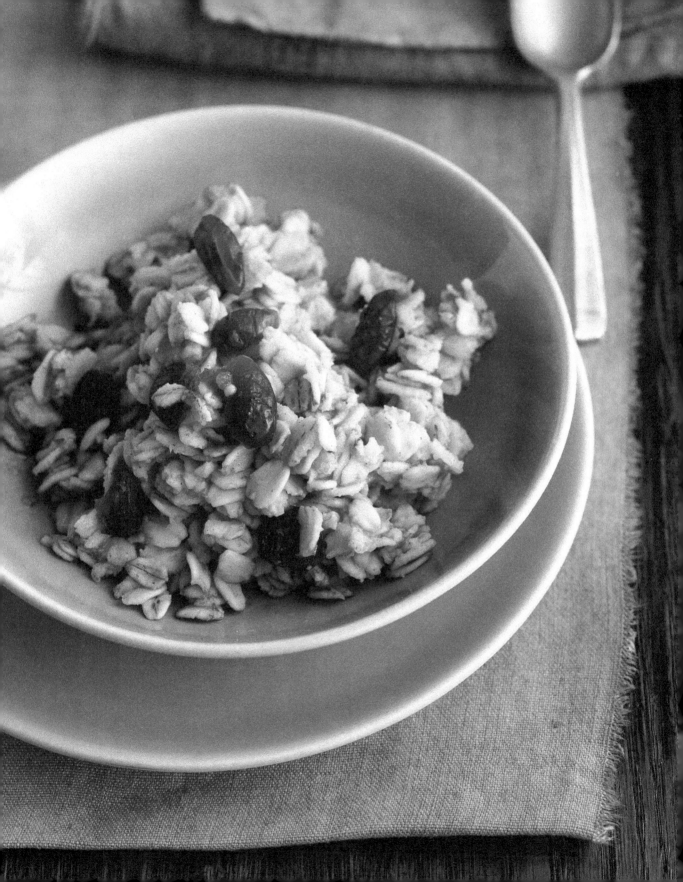

Oatmeal *with* Dried Cranberries

PREP TIME: 5 MINUTES / COOK TIME: 5 MINUTES

While this dish isn't included in the elimination phase of your GERD diet, if you find you aren't sensitive to dried fruits, this makes a hearty and delicious breakfast. The starch in the oats will absorb some of the acid from the dried fruit, so it shouldn't cause much acid. Serves 2

1 cup rolled oats

¾ cup water

¾ cup nonfat milk

¼ cup dried cranberries

1 teaspoon grated orange zest

Pinch salt

1   In a medium saucepan, bring the oats, water, milk, dried cranberries, orange zest, and salt to a rolling boil over high heat.

2   Reduce the heat to medium. Cook, stirring occasionally, for 5 minutes.

3   Remove the pan from the heat and let the oatmeal stand for 3 minutes before serving.

SUBSTITUTION TIP: *Dark or golden raisins also work well in this recipe.*

PER SERVING Calories: 197; Total Fat: 3g; Saturated Fat: 0g; Sodium: 131mg; Carbohydrates: 34g; Fiber: 5g; Protein: 8g

Zucchini and Mushroom Omelet

PREP TIME: 10 MINUTES / COOK TIME: 10 MINUTES

If you're looking for a heartier breakfast that will stick with you longer, then this easy omelet should fit the bill. The protein in the eggs will keep you going, while the zucchini and mushrooms add lots of flavor. Serves 2

2 tablespoons extra-virgin olive oil, divided

½ zucchini, peeled and chopped

2 ounces cremini mushrooms, sliced

½ teaspoon salt

½ teaspoon dried thyme

2 large eggs

4 large egg whites

¼ cup nonfat milk

1   In a large nonstick skillet, heat 1 tablespoon of olive oil over medium-high heat until it shimmers.

2   Add the zucchini, mushrooms, salt, and thyme and cook, stirring occasionally, until the vegetables have released their liquid and begin to brown, about 6 minutes. Remove the vegetables from the skillet and set aside.

3   While the vegetables cook, in a medium bowl whisk together the eggs, egg whites, and milk.

4   When the vegetables are done, heat the remaining 1 tablespoon of olive oil in the same nonstick skillet over medium-high heat until it shimmers.

5   Pour in the eggs and cook. As the eggs start to firm around the edges, use a spatula to carefully pull the edges away from the side of the pan. Tilt the pan to distribute any uncooked eggs into the spaces left by the edges you have pulled away. Cook until the eggs are firm, about 5 minutes.

6   Spoon the reserved zucchini and mushrooms over the eggs and fold the omelet over the filling.

7   Cut the omelet in half and serve.

INGREDIENT TIP: *For a little additional flavor, sprinkle 2 tablespoons of grated Parmesan cheese over the vegetables before folding the omelet. Avoid doing this during your two-week meal plan, however.*

PER SERVING Calories: 245; Total Fat: 19g; Saturated Fat: 3g; Sodium: 732mg; Carbohydrates: 5g; Fiber: 1g; Protein: 15g

Wild Mushroom Frittata *with* Herbs

PREP TIME: 10 MINUTES / COOK TIME: 15 MINUTES

A frittata is essentially an omelet that you finish in the oven. This one is chock-full of savory, meaty mushrooms and topped with fresh herbs, making it a satisfying and flavorful breakfast. Use a pan that transfers well from the stovetop to the oven. Serves 4

2 tablespoons extra-virgin olive oil

8 ounces cremini mushrooms, sliced

4 ounces enoki mushrooms, separated into individual mushrooms

4 large eggs

2 tablespoons nonfat milk

½ teaspoon salt

6 fresh basil leaves, cut into thin ribbons

1 tablespoon chopped fresh savory

1 tablespoon fresh thyme

1   Adjust the oven rack to the center position and preheat the broiler.

2   In an 8-inch ovenproof skillet, heat the olive oil over medium-high heat until it shimmers.

3   Add the mushrooms and cook, stirring occasionally, until browned, about 6 minutes.

4   In a small bowl, whisk together the eggs, milk, and salt.

5   Pour the egg mixture carefully over the mushrooms. Reduce the heat to medium. Cook undisturbed until the egg mixture solidifies around the edges, 2 to 3 minutes.

6   Use a rubber spatula to carefully pull the solid edges toward the center of the pan. Tilt the pan so the uncooked egg runs into the edges. Continue cooking until the edges solidify again, another minute or two.

7   Transfer the pan to the broiler and broil until the eggs set on the top, about 3 minutes.

8   Sprinkle the frittata with the basil, savory, and thyme. Cut into wedges and serve.

SUBSTITUTION TIP: *If you can't find enoki mushrooms, feel free to use any other type of mushrooms, such as chanterelles or oyster mushrooms, sliced.*

PER SERVING Calories: 303; Total Fat: 5g; Saturated Fat: 1g; Sodium: 104mg; Carbohydrates: 59g; Fiber: 2g; Protein: 7g

Pancakes *with* Sautéed Apples

PREP TIME: 10 MINUTES / COOK TIME: 20 MINUTES

These light, fluffy pancakes are the perfect base for sweet apples that have been spiced with cinnamon and ginger and mixed with a bit of honey. The result is a tasty breakfast that will give you energy for your day. Serves 4

For the apples

2 tablespoons unsalted butter

1 apple, cored and thinly sliced

½ teaspoon ground ginger

½ teaspoon ground cinnamon

2 tablespoons water

2 tablespoons honey

For the pancakes

1 cup all-purpose flour

1 tablespoon sugar

2 teaspoons baking powder

¼ teaspoon salt

1 cup nonfat milk

1 large egg, beaten

2 tablespoons extra-virgin olive oil

Nonstick cooking spray

For the apples

1   In a 12-inch nonstick skillet, heat the butter over medium-high heat until it bubbles.

2   Add the apple, ginger, and cinnamon and cook, stirring occasionally, until the apples soften and begin to brown, about 5 minutes.

3   Add the water and honey. Bring to a simmer and cook, stirring constantly, until the honey coats the apples. Cover and set aside.

For the pancakes

4   In a medium bowl, whisk together the flour, sugar, baking powder, and salt.

5   In another bowl, whisk together the milk, egg, and olive oil.

6   Add the wet ingredients to the dry ingredients, stirring until just mixed. There will be some streaks of flour left in the batter. ▸

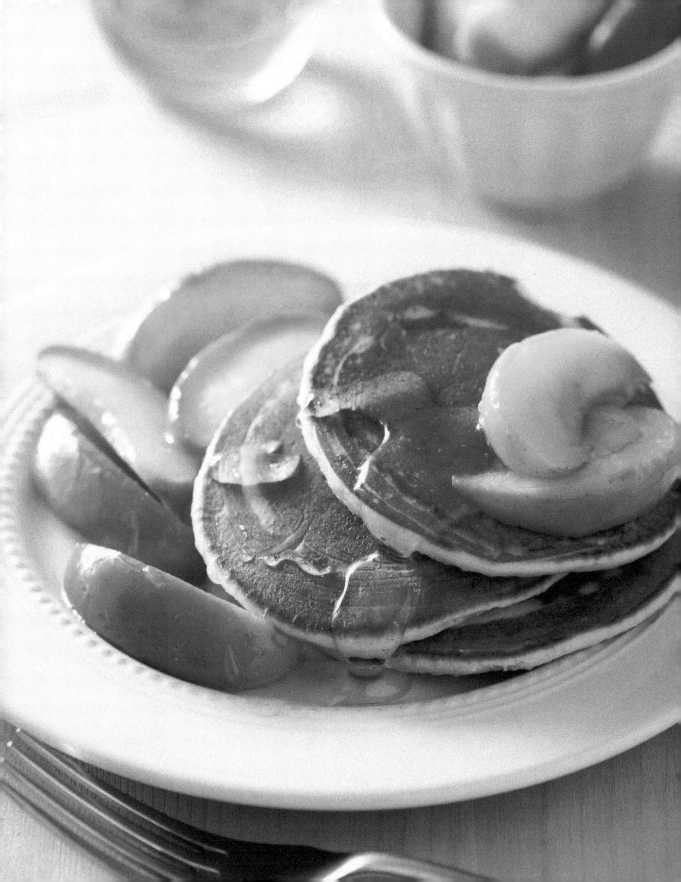

7   Heat a nonstick skillet over medium-high heat and spray with nonstick cooking spray.

8   Spoon about 3 tablespoons of batter per pancake into the heated skillet. Cook until the pancake batter bubbles on top, about 2 minutes.

9   Using a spatula, carefully flip the pancakes and cook on the second side until golden, about 2 minutes. Serve with the warm apples spooned on top.

SUBSTITUTION TIP: *You can replace the apples with thinly sliced pears and the cinnamon with nutmeg in this recipe, if you wish.*

PER SERVING Calories: 335; Total Fat: 14g; Saturated Fat: 5g; Sodium: 240mg; Carbohydrates: 46g; Fiber: 2g; Protein: 7g

Pumpkin Pancakes

Puréed pumpkin makes these pancakes moist and flavorful, while buttermilk gives them a tasty tang. You can substitute white whole-wheat flour for the all-purpose flour in this recipe, if you wish. Serves 4

1 cup all-purpose flour

1 tablespoon brown sugar

1½ teaspoons baking powder

¼ teaspoon ground ginger

¼ teaspoon ground nutmeg

Pinch salt

1 large egg, lightly beaten

¾ cup nonfat buttermilk

½ cup canned pumpkin purée

1 tablespoon extra-virgin olive oil

½ teaspoon alcohol-free vanilla

Nonstick cooking spray

½ cup pure maple syrup

1 In a medium bowl, whisk together the flour, brown sugar, baking powder, ginger, nutmeg, and salt.

2 In another bowl, whisk together the egg, buttermilk, pumpkin purée, olive oil, and vanilla.

3 Heat a nonstick skillet over medium-high heat. Spray it with nonstick cooking spray.

4 Pour a scant ¼ cup of batter into the pan for each pancake and cook until browned, about 4 minutes per side.

5 Serve topped with maple syrup.

INGREDIENT TIP: *Alcohol-free vanilla is available in the baking aisle at most grocery stores. Because it isn't technically vanilla extract, it is typically labeled alcohol-free vanilla flavor.*

PER SERVING Calories: 303; Total Fat: 5g; Saturated Fat: 1g; Sodium: 104mg; Carbohydrates: 59g; Fiber: 2g; Protein: 7g

Banana Crêpes

This recipe makes 12 crêpes. However, you'll only need 8 of the crêpes, so you can refrigerate or freeze the remaining 4 in a tightly sealed resealable bag for up to 1 week in the fridge or 6 months in the freezer. Then, when you want a quick breakfast, you can pull out the remaining crêpes and, if they're frozen, wrap them in a damp towel and microwave on low for 15 to 30 seconds per crêpe. Serves 4

1 cup plus 2 tablespoons all-purpose flour

Pinch salt

1 large egg, beaten

⅔ cup nonfat milk

Nonstick cooking spray

2 bananas, peeled and mashed lightly with a fork

1 cup plain nonfat yogurt

1 tablespoon honey

1 In a small bowl, whisk together the flour and salt.

2 In another bowl, whisk together the egg and milk.

3 Add the wet ingredients to the dry, whisking until completely smooth. Allow the batter to rest for 5 minutes.

4 Meanwhile, spray an 8-inch nonstick skillet with nonstick cooking spray and heat it over medium-high heat.

5 Pour a scant ¼ cup of batter into the skillet, swirling the skillet to distribute the batter evenly.

6 Cook for about 1 minute, using a spatula to lift the edges away from the bottom of the pan as they cook.

7 Flip the crêpe and cook on the other side for 30 seconds. Transfer the crêpe to a platter and cover to keep warm.

8 Repeat for the remaining crêpes, spraying the pan with more nonstick cooking spray between crêpes. Continue to stack the cooked crêpes on the platter.

9   When all of the crêpes are cooked, mix the mashed bananas, yogurt, and honey in a small bowl.

10 Wrap the crêpes around the banana filling and serve.

SUBSTITUTION TIP: *For dairy allergies, substitute rice milk for the milk and silken tofu for the yogurt. For wheat allergies or gluten intolerance, substitute sweet rice flour for the all-purpose flour.*

PER SERVING Calories: 271; Total Fat: 2g; Saturated Fat: 1g; Sodium: 120mg; Carbohydrates: 51g; Fiber: 3g; Protein: 11g

French Toast

If you like a little bit of citrus flavor without the burn, then this recipe is for you. Citrus zest flavors the custard for this French toast, giving you a hint of orange without the acid that comes from orange juice. Serves 4

2 large eggs, beaten

1 cup nonfat milk

½ teaspoon alcohol-free vanilla

Zest of ½ orange, grated

¼ teaspoon ground nutmeg

Pinch salt

4 slices whole-wheat bread

Nonstick cooking spray

½ cup pure maple syrup

1 In a small bowl, whisk together the eggs, milk, vanilla, orange zest, nutmeg, and salt.

2 Pour the mixture into a shallow pan.

3 Soak the bread slices in the egg mixture for 5 minutes, turning once.

4 While the bread soaks, preheat a large nonstick skillet over medium-high heat. Spray the skillet with nonstick cooking spray.

5 Cook the soaked bread in the preheated skillet until golden, 4 to 5 minutes per side.

6 Serve hot with the maple syrup.

WHY IT WORKS: *In traditional orange-flavored French toast, several items may trigger heartburn, including heavy cream, orange juice, and pure vanilla extract. This recipe calls for an alcohol-free version of vanilla. Removing the alcohol from the vanilla removes that acid reflux trigger. Likewise, citrus zest has plenty of citrus flavor without the acid inherent in the juice. Finally, replacing heavy cream with nonfat milk limits the fat for delicious, reflux-free French toast.*

PER SERVING Calories: 230; Total Fat: 3g; Saturated Fat: 1g; Sodium: 238mg; Carbohydrates: 42g; Fiber: 2g; Protein: 8g

Canadian Bacon
Breakfast Sandwich

PREP TIME: 15 MINUTES / COOK TIME: 10 MINUTES

A breakfast sandwich is a good portable breakfast that you can grab when you're in a hurry. This one is quick and easy, and you can take it with you to eat hot or cold. With all of the protein it contains, it's also a great way to start your day. Serves 1

1 whole-wheat English muffin, split

1 large egg

1 large egg white

¼ teaspoon salt

1 slice Canadian bacon

1   In a toaster, toast the English muffin to your desired doneness.

2   In a small bowl, whisk together the egg, egg white, and salt.

3   In a small nonstick skillet, cook the egg mixture over medium heat, stirring frequently, until done, about 4 minutes.

4   Place the eggs on one English muffin half.

5   Top with the Canadian bacon and the other muffin half and serve.

WHY IT WORKS: *Although ham and bacon tend to be fairly high in fat, Canadian bacon is relatively lean. Using just a small amount contributes plenty of flavor but a negligible amount of fat, leaving you with a satisfying, low-fat breakfast.*

PER SERVING Calories: 259; Total Fat: 8g; Saturated Fat: 2g; Sodium: 1,389mg; Carbohydrates: 28g; Fiber: 4g; Protein: 21g

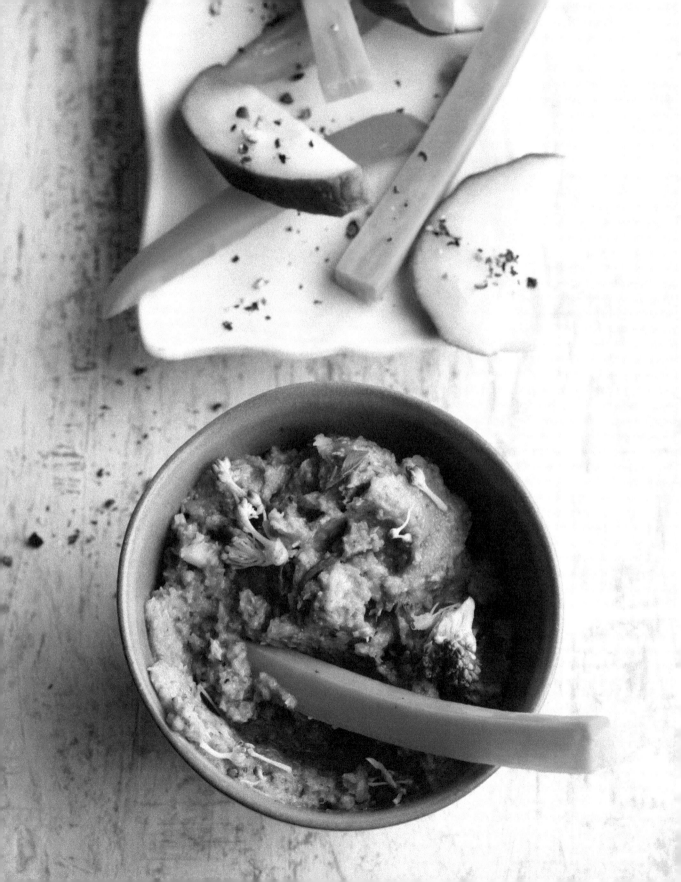

Chapter Five

Snacks and Appetizers

Apples *with* Honey-Yogurt Dip

PREP TIME: 5 MINUTES / COOK TIME: 0

If you're craving a quick snack, try these sliced apples dipped in a sweet, creamy yogurt sauce. You can mix it up quickly and be munching on a flavorful snack in just minutes. The dip will keep in an airtight container in the refrigerator for up to 4 days. Serves 2

½ cup plain nonfat yogurt

1 tablespoon honey

¼ teaspoon ground cinnamon

¼ teaspoon ground ginger

Pinch ground nutmeg

1 red apple, such as Fuji, cored and sliced

1   In a small bowl, whisk together the yogurt, honey, cinnamon, ginger, and nutmeg.

2   Serve in a small bowl with the sliced apples for dipping.

SUBSTITUTION TIP: *For people with dairy allergies, you can replace the non-fat yogurt with plain low-fat soy yogurt. You can also replace the ground ginger with grated fresh ginger if you wish.*

PER SERVING Calories: 125; Total Fat: 1g; Saturated Fat: 1g; Sodium: 44mg; Carbohydrates: 26g; Fiber: 2g; Protein: 4g

Spinach Dip

Nonfat sour cream adds a tangy flavor to this tasty spinach dip. Serve it alongside carrot or celery sticks, or spread it on low-fat whole-grain crackers for a quick and fortifying snack. The dip will keep well in an airtight container in the refrigerator for up to 1 week. Serves 4

2 cups frozen spinach, thawed

2 cups nonfat sour cream

Zest of ½ lemon, grated

½ teaspoon salt

¼ teaspoon ground nutmeg

Pinch ground cloves

1   In a colander, drain the thawed spinach, pressing on it with a spoon to remove any excess water.

2   In a small bowl, whisk together the sour cream, lemon zest, salt, nutmeg, and cloves.

3   Stir in the spinach. Serve cold.

SUBSTITUTION TIP: *If you're allergic to dairy, you can put 1 cup of silken tofu in a blender and blend until the tofu resembles sour cream. Thin with a little water if necessary.*

PER SERVING Calories: 130; Total Fat: 0g; Saturated Fat: 0g; Sodium: 430mg; Carbohydrates: 22g; Fiber: 1g; Protein: 5g

Broccoli Dip *with* Vegetables

PREP TIME: 10 MINUTES / COOK TIME: 5 MINUTES

Get a double helping of vegetables and fiber by dipping carrot sticks or zucchini rounds into this tasty broccoli dip. Nonfat Greek yogurt makes it creamy, giving it a smooth mouthfeel, while fresh herbs add loads of flavor. Serves 4

1 cup broccoli florets

1 cup plain nonfat Greek yogurt

1 teaspoon chopped fresh dill

1 teaspoon fresh thyme

1 tablespoon grated lemon zest

½ teaspoon salt

4 carrots, peeled and cut into sticks

1   In a saucepan fitted with a steamer basket and lid, steam the broccoli over boiling water for 5 minutes. Rinse under cold water to stop the cooking.

2   In the bowl of a blender or food processor, combine the yogurt, cooled broccoli, dill, thyme, lemon zest, and salt. Blend until puréed.

3   Serve with the carrot sticks for dipping.

SUBSTITUTION TIP: *This recipe also works with other cruciferous vegetables in place of the broccoli, including cauliflower and broccolini. Both have a milder flavor than the broccoli.*

PER SERVING Calories: 68; Total Fat: 0g; Saturated Fat: 0g; Sodium: 386mg; Carbohydrates: 13g; Fiber: 3g; Protein: 4g

Sweet and Spicy Popcorn

PREP TIME: 5 MINUTES / COOK TIME: 0

This popcorn will bring a little sweetness to your day, with tasty, sweet kernels tossed with fragrant spices. Use an air popper to pop the corn so that you don't have to add oil. You can take this snack with you in a tightly sealed bag or container. Serves 2

2 tablespoons brown sugar

½ teaspoon ground cinnamon

½ teaspoon ground allspice

¼ teaspoon ground ginger

4 cups air-popped popcorn

1   In a small bowl, combine the brown sugar, cinnamon, allspice, and ginger until well mixed.

2   In a large bowl, toss the popcorn with the brown sugar mixture. Serve warm or at room temperature.

SUBSTITUTION TIP: *If you prefer savory popcorn to sweet, omit the brown sugar, cinnamon, allspice, and ginger. Instead, make your spice mixture from 2 tablespoons of Italian seasoning and 1 teaspoon of salt.*

PER SERVING Calories: 99; Total Fat: 1g; Saturated Fat: 0g; Sodium: 4mg; Carbohydrates: 22g; Fiber: 3g; Protein: 2g

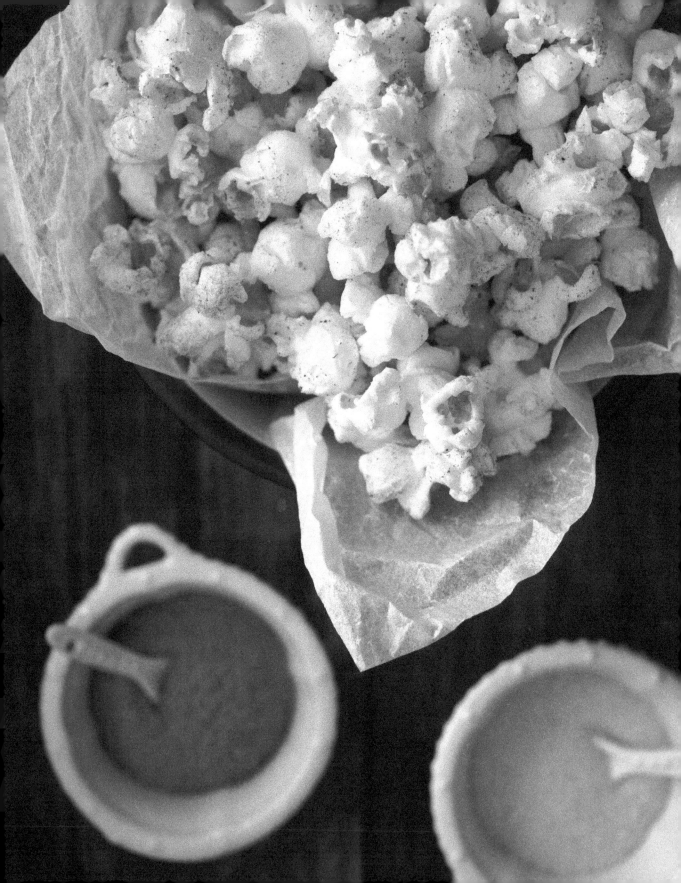

Cinnamon-Sugar Popcorn

PREP TIME: 5 MINUTES / COOK TIME: 0

Sometimes simple is best, and this sweet popcorn delivers. It brings back memories of cinnamon toast in childhood, and it's deliciously simple to make. The recipe calls for a tablespoon of butter to help the cinnamon and sugar stick to the popcorn, but you can leave it out if you wish. Serves 2

¼ cup sugar

1 teaspoon ground cinnamon

1 tablespoon unsalted butter, melted

4 cups air-popped popcorn

1   In a small bowl, combine the sugar and cinnamon.

2   In a large bowl, toss the popcorn with the butter, and then add the cinnamon-sugar mixture. Serve warm or at room temperature.

SUBSTITUTION TIP: *To cut down on fat, try spraying the popcorn with a popcorn spray instead of using butter to help the cinnamon and sugar mixture stick.*

PER SERVING Calories: 209; Total Fat: 6g; Saturated Fat: 4g; Sodium: 42mg; Carbohydrates: 38g; Fiber: 3g; Protein: 2g

Stuffed Mushroom Caps

PREP TIME: 15 MINUTES / COOK TIME: 25 MINUTES

This is another delicious party appetizer, or a great snack. Use medium-size cremini mushrooms, and reserve the stems to put into the stuffing. Bread crumbs add a nice crunch. Serves 4

12 cremini mushrooms, cleaned

2 tablespoons extra-virgin olive oil

2 cups baby spinach, chopped

Zest of ½ orange, grated

1 teaspoon dried thyme

½ teaspoon salt

¼ teaspoon ground nutmeg

¼ cup bread crumbs

1   Preheat the oven to 350°F.

2   Line a baking sheet with parchment paper or aluminum foil.

3   Remove the mushroom stems and chop the stems into fine dice.

4   In a medium skillet, heat the olive oil over medium-high heat until it shimmers.

5   Add the chopped mushroom stems and cook, stirring occasionally, until browned and soft, about 5 minutes.

6   Add the spinach and cook, stirring occasionally, until the spinach is wilted, 3 to 4 minutes. Remove from the heat and stir in the orange zest, thyme, salt, and nutmeg.

7   Place the mushroom caps on the lined baking sheet with the tops down. Stuff the mushroom and spinach mixture into the caps, and sprinkle with the bread crumbs.

8   Bake until the bread crumbs brown and the mushrooms are soft, about 15 minutes. Serve warm.

INGREDIENT TIP: *Mushrooms are like little sponges, so if you wash them, they'll soak up all of the water and grow soggy. Instead, use a soft brush or a paper towel to wipe away any dirt.*

PER SERVING Calories: 108; Total Fat: 8g; Saturated Fat: 1g; Sodium: 356mg; Carbohydrates: 8g; Fiber: 1g; Protein: 3g

Baked Sweet Potato Chips

PREP TIME: 10 MINUTES / COOK TIME: 55 MINUTES

While these chips take a little bit of time in the oven to crisp up, your active work time is hardly anything at all. The low temperature of the oven dehydrates the chips, making them crispy without adding any fat. Try them with the Spinach Dip (page 83). Serves 2

1 sweet potato, scrubbed   1 teaspoon salt

1   Preheat the oven to 200°F.

2   Line two large baking sheets with parchment paper or aluminum foil.

3   Using a very sharp knife, slice the sweet potatoes into very thin slices. Arrange them in a single layer on the lined baking sheets.

4   Sprinkle the chips evenly with the salt.

5   Bake until the chips are crispy, 50 to 55 minutes. Serve.

COOKING TIP: *If you have a mandolin or a food processor with a slicing blade, use one of these tools to quickly and evenly slice the potato.*

PER SERVING Calories: 52; Total Fat: 0g; Saturated Fat: 0g; Sodium: 1,183mg; Carbohydrates: 12g; Fiber: 2g; Protein: 1g

Potato Pancakes *with* Herbed Sour Cream

PREP TIME: 10 MINUTES / COOK TIME: 20 MINUTES

These potato pancakes make a delicious snack or appetizer. Try them topped with smoked salmon or shrimp salad, which transforms them from an appetizer to a tasty meal. Serves 4

2 russet potatoes, peeled and grated

1 large egg, beaten

2 tablespoons all-purpose flour

½ teaspoon salt

2 tablespoons extra-virgin olive oil

2 tablespoons chopped fresh thyme

¼ cup nonfat sour cream

1   In a large bowl, stir together the grated potatoes, egg, flour, and salt until well mixed.

2   Heat a nonstick skillet over medium-high heat. Add the olive oil and heat until it shimmers.

3   Spoon about ¼ cup of batter per pancake into the skillet. Cook until golden brown, about 5 minutes per side.

4   In a small bowl, stir the thyme into the sour cream.

5   Serve the hot pancakes with a dollop of the sour cream.

SUBSTITUTION TIP: *This recipe works well with grated sweet potatoes as well. Try them topped with the Applesauce with Fennel and Ginger (page 199).*

PER SERVING Calories: 182; Total Fat: 8g; Saturated Fat: 1g; Sodium: 326mg; Carbohydrates: 23g; Fiber: 3g; Protein: 4g

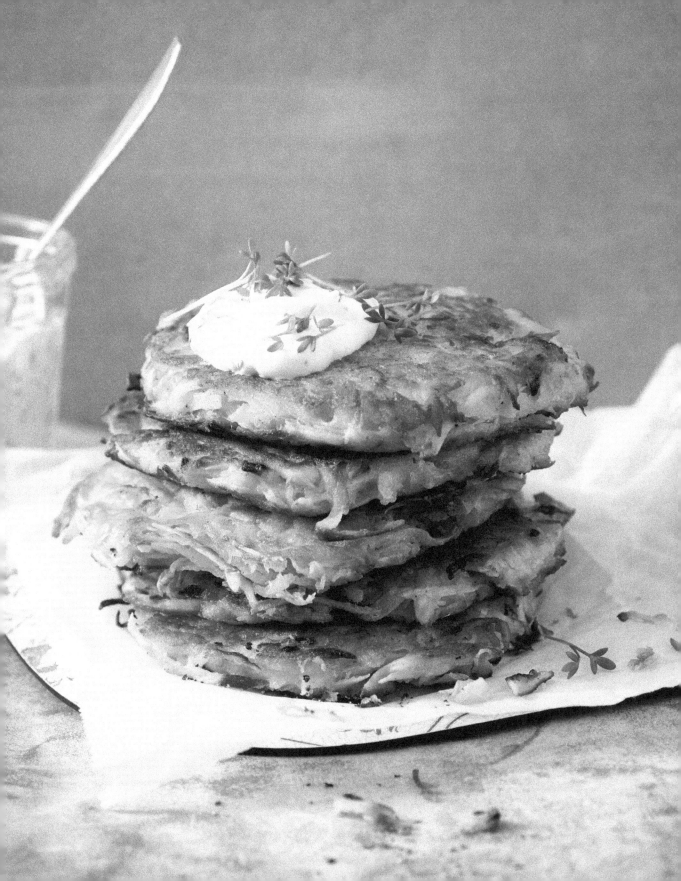

Zucchini and Smoked Salmon Rounds

PREP TIME: 10 MINUTES / COOK TIME: 0

Perfect for a party, this canapé-style appetizer combines the savory flavor of smoked salmon with tangy yogurt and tarragon. Tarragon is an ideal accompaniment for seafood, because its mild licorice-like flavor complements the sweetness of the fish. For a party, double or triple the recipe. Serves 4

1 cup plain nonfat Greek yogurt

2 tablespoons chopped fresh tarragon

Zest of ½ lemon, grated

6 ounces smoked salmon, flaked

1 medium zucchini, sliced

1   In a small bowl, combine the yogurt, tarragon, and lemon zest until well mixed.

2   Fold in the salmon.

3   Spoon the mixture onto the zucchini slices and serve.

SUBSTITUTION TIP: *If you can't find fresh tarragon, or you don't like it, then substitute chopped fresh dill instead. Dill also works very well with smoked salmon.*

PER SERVING Calories: 93; Total Fat: 2g; Saturated Fat: 0g; Sodium: 901mg; Carbohydrates: 7g; Fiber: 1g; Protein: 12g

Shrimp Salad *on* Melba Toast

PREP TIME: 15 MINUTES / COOK TIME: 0

Melba toast offers plenty of crunch without a lot of fat, so it's the perfect base for this appetizer or snack. The shrimp salad uses baby shrimp, which you can find precooked at the grocery store seafood counter. Serves 4

½ cup plain nonfat Greek yogurt

3 tablespoons chopped fresh cilantro, plus more for garnish

1 teaspoon grated lime zest

½ teaspoon salt

8 ounces cooked baby shrimp

1 celery stalk, finely chopped

8 pieces melba toast

1   In a small bowl, whisk together the yogurt, chopped cilantro, lime zest, and salt.

2   Stir in the shrimp and celery.

3   Spoon the mixture onto the melba toasts.

4   Garnish with additional cilantro and serve.

SUBSTITUTION TIP: *If you have a shellfish allergy, you can replace the shrimp with flaked fish, such as halibut or salmon.*

PER SERVING Calories: 128; Total Fat: 1g; Saturated Fat: 0g; Sodium: 541mg; Carbohydrates: 12g; Fiber: 1g; Protein: 16g

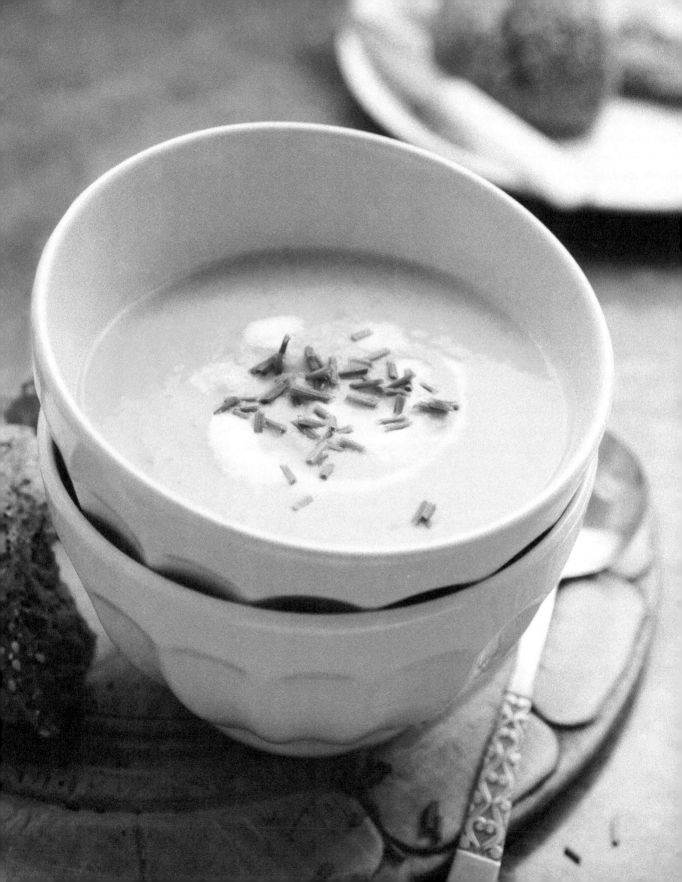

Chapter Six

Side Dishes

Creamed Spinach

PREP TIME: 5 MINUTES / COOK TIME: 5 MINUTES

This quick and satisfying side dish features healthy spinach in a creamy sauce. Traditional creamed spinach is high in fat, but this version uses nonfat milk and eliminates the cheese. Serves 4

2 tablespoons extra-virgin
olive oil, divided

12 ounces spinach, stems removed

1 tablespoon all-purpose flour

½ cup nonfat milk

¼ teaspoon salt

⅛ teaspoon ground nutmeg

1   In a large skillet, heat 1 tablespoon of olive oil over medium-high heat until it shimmers.

2   Add the spinach and cook, stirring occasionally, until it wilts, about 2 minutes. Remove from the heat and set aside.

3   In a small saucepan, heat the remaining 1 tablespoon of olive oil over medium-high heat until it shimmers. Stir in the flour and cook, stirring constantly, for 1 minute.

4   Stir in the milk, salt, and nutmeg and cook, whisking constantly, until the mixture thickens, about 1 minute.

5   Stir the spinach into the white sauce and serve hot.

INGREDIENT TIP: *Spinach can be pretty gritty with dirt. The best way to wash it is in a bowl filled with water. Gently agitate the spinach with your hands. Drain the water and rinse the bowl. Repeat this process until no dirt falls into the bottom of the bowl after you agitate the spinach. Pat it dry with paper towels.*

PER SERVING Calories: 98; Total Fat: 7g; Saturated Fat: 1g; Sodium: 231mg; Carbohydrates: 6g; Fiber: 2g; Protein: 4g

Creamy Pumpkin Soup

PREP TIME: 5 MINUTES / COOK TIME: 10 MINUTES

This simple soup doesn't have many ingredients, but it is so satisfying. Serve it as a side dish, an appetizer, or even a simple lunch or dinner. You'll enjoy both the simplicity required to make it, and its hearty flavor. Serves 4

2 cups canned pumpkin purée

2 cups Chicken Broth (page 185)

1 cup light coconut milk

1 tablespoon pure maple syrup

½ teaspoon salt

1 tablespoon chopped fresh chives

1   In a large saucepan, combine the pumpkin purée, chicken broth, coconut milk, syrup, and salt. Cook over medium-high heat, stirring occasionally, until heated through, about 10 minutes.

2   Sprinkle with the chives just before serving.

SUBSTITUTION TIP: *While this contains such a small amount of chives that they shouldn't aggravate your GERD, if you are especially sensitive, then you may replace the chives with 2 tablespoons of chopped fresh thyme. It will have an earthier flavor while still offering the sparkle of fresh herbs.*

PER SERVING Calories: 108; Total Fat: 4g; Saturated Fat: 3g; Sodium: 694mg; Carbohydrates: 16g; Fiber: 4g; Protein: 5g

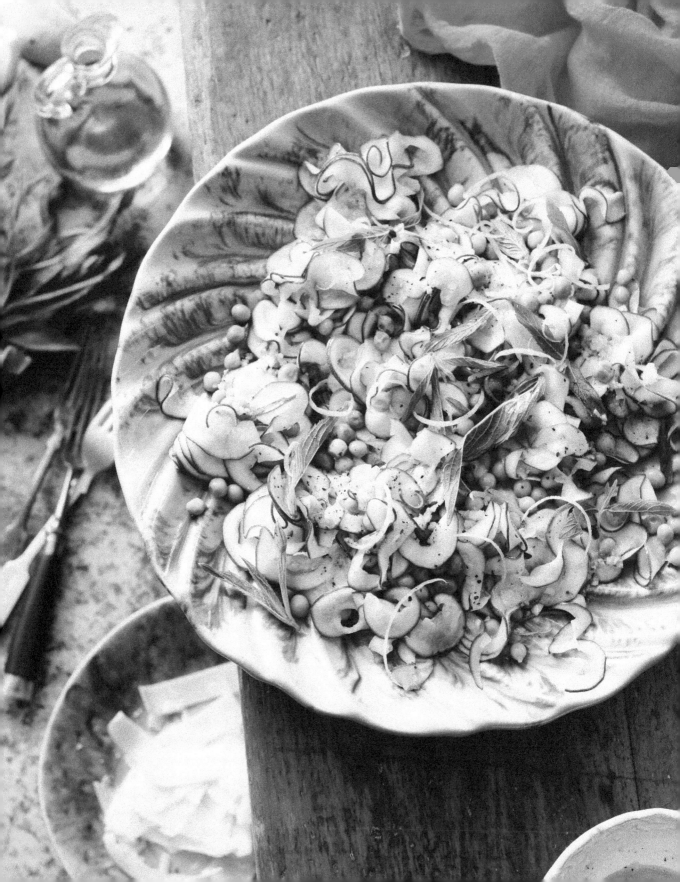

Zucchini Strips *with* Peas

PREP TIME: 10 MINUTES / COOK TIME: 5 MINUTES

This simple sauté is vividly green and fresh with the flavors of sweet peas and rosemary. It is also very quick to cook, because you cut the zucchini into thin strips that warm up quickly. It refrigerates well, so it makes for great leftovers. Serves 4

2 tablespoons extra-virgin olive oil

2 medium zucchini, cut into strips with a vegetable peeler

1 cup peas (fresh or frozen)

2 tablespoons chopped fresh rosemary

1 teaspoon grated lemon zest

½ teaspoon salt

1   In a large skillet, heat the olive oil over medium-high heat until it shimmers.

2   Add the zucchini, peas, rosemary, lemon zest, and salt.

3   Cook, stirring frequently, until the vegetables are soft, about 5 minutes. Serve warm.

INGREDIENT TIP: *If you aren't sensitive, you can sprinkle the zucchini and peas with ¼ cup of Parmesan cheese just before serving.*

PER SERVING Calories: 111; Total Fat: 8g; Saturated Fat: 1g; Sodium: 303mg; Carbohydrates: 10g; Fiber: 4g; Protein: 3g

Honey-Roasted Asparagus

PREP TIME: 5 MINUTES / COOK TIME: 30 MINUTES

Sweet honey complements the grassy flavor of asparagus. Roasting adds a rich depth of flavor to the tender spears, making the flavor more interesting than if you were to steam the vegetable. This is a delicious side dish with fish. Serves 4

1 tablespoon extra-virgin olive oil

2 tablespoons honey

½ teaspoon salt

1 pound asparagus, trimmed

1   Preheat the oven to 375°F.

2   In a large bowl, whisk together the olive oil, honey, and salt.

3   Add the asparagus and toss to combine.

4   Place the asparagus in a single layer in a roasting pan.

5   Roast until the asparagus is soft and beginning to brown, 25 to 30 minutes. Serve warm.

INGREDIENT TIP: *When preparing asparagus, you need to remove the thick stems from the bottom of the stalks. To do this, hold the asparagus spears at both ends and bend lightly until the stalk snaps. Discard the fibrous ends.*

PER SERVING Calories: 85; Total Fat: 4g; Saturated Fat: 1g; Sodium: 293mg; Carbohydrates: 13g; Fiber: 2g; Protein: 3g

Smoky Baked Beans

PREP TIME: 10 MINUTES / COOK TIME: 1 HOUR AND 10 MINUTES

These baked beans take about an hour to cook in the oven, but you'll spend only about 10 minutes fussing over them. Liquid smoke is the key to their wonderfully smoky flavor. You can find it in the seasoning aisle of the grocery store. Serves 8

2 tablespoons extra-virgin olive oil

1 celery stalk, finely chopped

1 carrot, finely chopped

1 tablespoon all-purpose flour

1 cup Chicken Broth (page 185)

1 (14-ounce) can navy beans, rinsed and drained

2 tablespoons brown sugar

2 tablespoons soy sauce

1 tablespoon Dijon mustard

¼ teaspoon liquid smoke

1 teaspoon salt

1   Preheat the oven to 350°F.

2   In a large skillet, heat the olive oil over medium-high heat until it shimmers.

3   Add the celery and carrot and cook, stirring occasionally, until soft and starting to brown, about 5 minutes.

4   Add the flour and cook, stirring constantly, for 1 minute.

5   Add the chicken broth and cook, stirring constantly, until it thickens, 1 to 2 minutes more.

6   Stir in the navy beans, brown sugar, soy sauce, mustard, liquid smoke, and salt. Bring to a simmer, stirring constantly.

7   Pour the bean mixture into a 9-inch square baking pan. Bake until bubbly and hot, about 1 hour. Serve.

INGREDIENT TIP: *A little liquid smoke goes a long way. If you prefer your beans smokier, taste them before baking, and add more if desired.*

PER SERVING Calories: 221; Total Fat: 5g; Saturated Fat: 1g; Sodium: 659mg; Carbohydrates: 34g; Fiber: 13g; Protein: 12g

Loaded Mashed Potatoes

PREP TIME: 10 MINUTES / COOK TIME: 10 MINUTES

Mashed potatoes are a favorite side dish of many, but often they are laden with fat that can trigger acid reflux. This version uses chicken broth to up the flavor and eliminates the fatty butter. Nonfat sour cream adds tang and makes the potatoes really creamy. Serves 4

2 russet potatoes, peeled and cut into 1-inch pieces

½ cup Chicken Broth (page 185)

½ cup nonfat sour cream

½ teaspoon salt

4 slices turkey bacon, browned and crumbled

1 Put the potatoes in a medium saucepan and cover with water. Bring the water to a boil over medium-high heat.

2 Cook until the potatoes are tender, about 10 minutes. Drain the potatoes in a colander.

3 Return the potatoes to the saucepan and mash them with a potato masher until smooth.

4 Stir in the chicken broth, sour cream, and salt until well blended.

5 Stir in the turkey bacon. Serve hot.

COOKING TIP: *For fluffier mashed potatoes, use a potato ricer, which you can find in cooking supply stores. Put the cooked and drained potatoes through the ricer into a bowl. Then, in a small bowl, mix the chicken broth, sour cream, and salt until well combined. Stir them into the potatoes, and then add the bacon.*

PER SERVING Calories: 160; Total Fat: 7g; Saturated Fat: 4g; Sodium: 528mg; Carbohydrates: 18g; Fiber: 3g; Protein: 6g

Baked Butternut Squash

PREP TIME: 15 MINUTES / COOK TIME: 30 MINUTES

Butternut squash is sweet and earthy. It's a great accompaniment to meat and poultry dishes. This version is lightly dusted with cinnamon and then roasted to a sweet golden brown in the oven. Serves 4

1 butternut squash, peeled and cut into 1-inch cubes

1 tablespoon extra-virgin olive oil

2 tablespoons brown sugar

1 teaspoon ground cinnamon

½ teaspoon salt

¼ teaspoon ground nutmeg

1 Preheat the oven to 400°F.

2 Put the squash cubes in a large bowl and drizzle them with the olive oil, tossing to coat.

3 In a small bowl, whisk together the brown sugar, cinnamon, salt, and nutmeg.

4 Toss the spice mixture with the squash.

5 Place the squash on a large baking sheet in a single layer.

6 Bake until the squash is tender and begins to brown, about 30 minutes. Serve warm.

SUBSTITUTION TIP: *This recipe will also work with sweet potatoes or acorn squash if you are unable to find butternut squash.*

PER SERVING Calories: 81; Total Fat: 4g; Saturated Fat: 1g; Sodium: 295mg; Carbohydrates: 13g; Fiber: 2g; Protein: 1g

Rice *with* Peas, Green Beans, and Carrots

PREP TIME: 10 MINUTES / COOK TIME: 15 MINUTES

Rice makes a filling and nourishing side dish. Here, when it's paired with deeply browned vegetables and flavorful herbs, it is even more satisfying. Use precooked rice to save time with this dish. Serves 4

4 ounces green beans, trimmed

2 tablespoons extra-virgin olive oil

1 large carrot, peeled and thinly sliced

1 cup peas (fresh or frozen)

4 ounces cremini mushrooms, thinly sliced

1 teaspoon salt

¼ cup Chicken Broth (page 185)

1 cup cooked brown rice

2 tablespoons chopped fresh tarragon

1   Bring a large pot of water to a boil over medium-high heat. Add the beans and cook for 3 minutes. Drain the beans.

2   In a large skillet, heat the olive oil over medium-high heat until it shimmers.

3   Add the cooked beans, carrot, peas, mushrooms, and salt and cook, stirring occasionally, until the vegetables begin to brown, about 7 minutes.

4   Add the chicken broth and use the side of the spoon to scrape any browned bits from the bottom of the pan.

5   Stir in the rice. Cook, stirring frequently, until the rice is heated through and the liquid absorbed, 3 to 4 minutes.

6   Stir in the tarragon just before serving.

SUBSTITUTION TIP: *You can replace the rice in this dish with an equal amount of cooked orzo. Orzo is a rice-shaped pasta that has a slightly nuttier flavor than rice.*

PER SERVING Calories: 290; Total Fat: 9g; Saturated Fat: 1g; Sodium: 649mg; Carbohydrates: 47g; Fiber: 5g; Protein: 7g

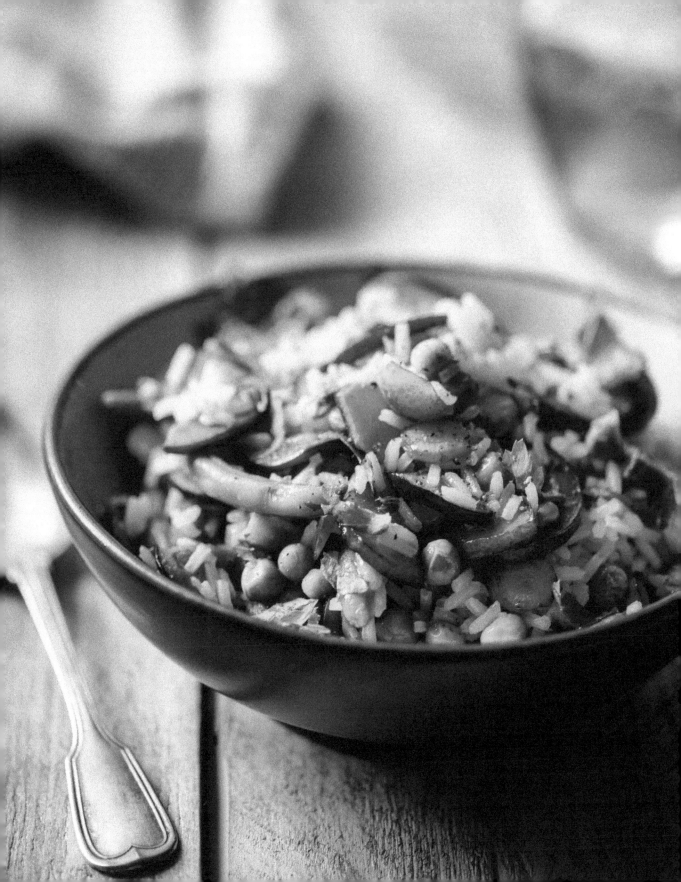

Green Bean Casserole

PREP TIME: 10 MINUTES / COOK TIME: 40 MINUTES

This warm, bubbly casserole is a favorite at holiday meals, but it's traditionally a big pan of heartburn waiting to happen. This version removes all of the heartburn hazards, providing you with a tasty casserole that won't leave you reaching for antacids. Serves 8

12 ounces green beans, trimmed

2 tablespoons extra-virgin olive oil, divided

4 ounces button mushrooms, sliced

1 tablespoon all-purpose flour

1 cup nonfat milk

½ cup nonfat sour cream

1 tablespoon soy sauce

1 teaspoon dried thyme

½ teaspoon salt

¼ cup bread crumbs

1　Preheat the oven to 350°F.

2　Fill a large pot with water and bring to a boil over high heat.

3　Add the green beans and cook until they are soft, about 5 minutes. Drain in a colander and set aside.

4　In a large skillet, heat 1 tablespoon of olive oil over medium-high heat until it shimmers.

5　Add the mushrooms and cook, stirring occasionally, until they are browned, about 5 minutes. Remove from the pan and set aside.

6　In the same skillet, add the remaining 1 tablespoon of olive oil, heating it until it shimmers.

7　Add the flour and cook, stirring constantly, for 1 minute.

8　Add the milk and cook, stirring constantly, until it thickens, about 1 minute more.

9　Stir in the sour cream, soy sauce, thyme, and salt.

10　Bring to a simmer, and stir in the cooked beans and mushrooms.

11 Transfer the mixture to a 9-inch square baking pan. Top with the bread crumbs.

12 Bake until the bread crumbs brown and the beans are bubbly, about 25 minutes. Serve.

INGREDIENT TIP: *To prepare the beans, trim the ends and then cut them in half crosswise. You can also substitute one 14-ounce can of drained beans in this recipe. If you do, there's no need to boil them.*

PER SERVING Calories: 107; Total Fat: 7g; Saturated Fat: 2g; Sodium: 312mg; Carbohydrates: 9g; Fiber: 2g; Protein: 3g

Creamy Mushroom Rice

PREP TIME: 15 MINUTES, PLUS 1 TO 2 HOURS FOR MUSHROOMS TO STEEP / COOK TIME: 45 MINUTES

There's something that's just so satisfying and warming about rice, particularly in this dish. It gets its flavor from soaking dried mushrooms in chicken broth and its creaminess from nonfat sour cream. It makes a great side dish for poultry. Serves 6

1½ cups Chicken Broth (page 185)

2 ounces dried mushrooms

1 tablespoon extra-virgin olive oil

4 ounces cremini mushrooms, sliced

1 cup brown rice

½ teaspoon fish sauce

1 teaspoon dried thyme

½ cup nonfat sour cream

¼ cup nonfat milk

1   In a small saucepan, bring the chicken broth to a simmer over medium heat.

2   Remove the pan from the heat and add the dried mushrooms. Cover the pan and allow the mushrooms to steep for 1 to 2 hours.

3   In a medium saucepan, heat the olive oil over medium-high heat until it shimmers.

4   Add the cremini mushrooms and cook, stirring occasionally, until browned, about 5 minutes.

5   Remove the browned mushrooms from the pan and set aside.

6   When the soaked mushrooms are soft, remove them from the broth (reserve the broth) and chop them. Pour the broth and the dried mushrooms into the same saucepan. Add the rice, fish sauce, and thyme.

7   Bring the mixture to a simmer over medium-high heat. Reduce the heat to medium, cover, and cook for 40 minutes.

8   Turn the heat off and allow the rice to sit for 10 minutes, covered. Then uncover and fluff the rice with a fork.

9   Place the rice over low heat and stir in the sour cream, milk, and reserved cremini mushrooms. Cook, stirring constantly, until heated through, about 3 minutes. Serve warm.

INGREDIENT TIP: *If you can find them, dried porcini mushrooms are the most flavorful. However, if you can't find them, then use any dried mushrooms, such as shiitakes.*

PER SERVING Calories: 197; Total Fat: 8g; Saturated Fat: 3g; Sodium: 248mg; Carbohydrates: 27g; Fiber: 1g; Protein: 5g

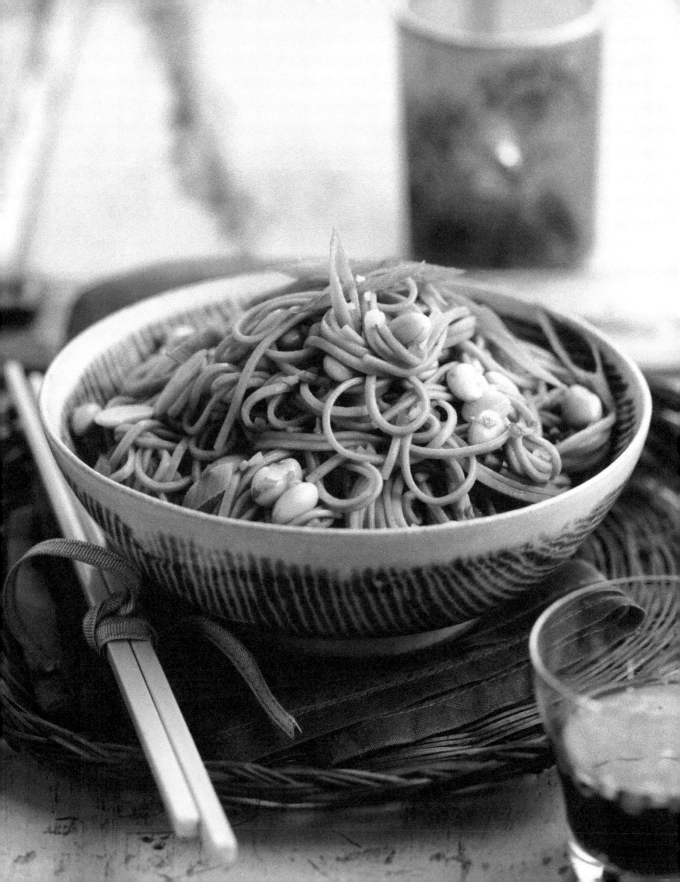

Chapter Seven

Vegetarian and Vegan

Carrot and Ginger Soup

PREP TIME: 5 MINUTES / COOK TIME: 30 MINUTES

Carrots and ginger are a classic flavor combination that comes together beautifully in this satisfying soup. The soup freezes and refrigerates well, so it's a great make-ahead meal that you can take for lunches during the week. Serves 4

4½ cups Vegetable Broth (page 184)

4 cups peeled and diced carrots

¼ cup finely diced fresh ginger

2 tablespoons soy sauce

½ teaspoon salt

¼ teaspoon ground nutmeg

1   In a large pot, combine all of the ingredients. Bring to a simmer over medium-high heat.

2   Cover and simmer until the carrots are soft, about 30 minutes.

3   Pour the soup into a blender (you may need to work in batches) and purée until smooth. Serve.

COOKING TIP: *When puréeing hot food in a blender, be sure to let steam escape occasionally so pressure does not build up. To safely do this, remove the insert in the lid and cover the hole with a kitchen towel.*

PER SERVING Calories: 112; Total Fat: 2g; Saturated Fat: 1g; Sodium: 1,678mg; Carbohydrates: 16g; Fiber: 4g; Protein: 7g

Creamy Asparagus Soup

PREP TIME: 5 MINUTES / COOK TIME: 15 MINUTES

This soup tastes best in the early spring when asparagus is in season. The tender, slightly sweet asparagus makes a satisfying and flavorful soup that works well for lunch or dinner. It will keep in the refrigerator, in an airtight container, for up to 1 week. Serves 4

2 pounds asparagus, trimmed

1 tablespoon extra-virgin olive oil

2 tablespoons all-purpose flour

2 cups nonfat milk

1 teaspoon dried tarragon

1 teaspoon salt

1   Bring a large pot of water to a boil over medium-high heat.

2   Cut the trimmed asparagus into 1-inch pieces and add them to the pot of boiling water.

3   Cover and simmer until the asparagus is soft, about 10 minutes. Drain the asparagus in a colander.

4   In a large saucepan, heat the olive oil over medium-high heat until it shimmers.

5   Stir in the flour and cook, stirring constantly, for 1 minute.

6   Stir in the milk, tarragon, and salt. Cook, stirring constantly, until the mixture thickens, 2 to 3 minutes.

7   Put the drained asparagus in the blender with the milk mixture and purée until smooth. Be sure to remove the insert in the blender lid and cover the hole with a kitchen towel to allow steam to escape while puréeing. Serve.

SUBSTITUTION TIP: *You can make this creamy asparagus soup vegan by replacing the nonfat milk with low-fat soymilk.*

PER SERVING Calories: 135; Total Fat: 4g; Saturated Fat: 1g; Sodium: 651mg; Carbohydrates: 18g; Fiber: 5g; Protein: 9g

Smoky Black Bean Soup

PREP TIME: 10 MINUTES / COOK TIME: 15 MINUTES

This is a hearty soup that is delicious for lunch or dinner. It freezes well as long as it is tightly sealed. You can keep it in the freezer for up to 6 months, so consider making a double batch so you'll have food ready for those days when you just don't feel like cooking. Serves 6

1 tablespoon extra-virgin olive oil

2 carrots, peeled and finely chopped

1 celery stalk, finely chopped

1 (14-ounce) can black beans, rinsed and drained

3 cups Vegetable Broth (page 184)

2 tablespoons soy sauce

2 tablespoons brown sugar

1 teaspoon ground cumin

½ teaspoon liquid smoke

Zest of 1 lime, grated

¼ cup chopped fresh cilantro

½ avocado, cubed, for garnish

¼ cup nonfat sour cream, for garnish

1   In a large pot, heat the olive oil over medium-high heat until it shimmers.

2   Add the carrots and celery and cook, stirring occasionally, until browned, 5 to 7 minutes.

3   Add the black beans, vegetable broth, soy sauce, brown sugar, cumin, liquid smoke, and lime zest. Bring to a simmer and cook, stirring occasionally, until the vegetables are soft, about 10 minutes.

4   Stir in the cilantro.

5   Transfer the mixture to a blender and purée until smooth. Be sure to remove the insert in the blender lid and cover the hole with a kitchen towel to allow steam to escape while puréeing.

6   Serve hot, garnished with the avocado and a dollop of sour cream.

SUBSTITUTION TIP: *For a dairy-free, vegan version, simply omit the sour cream altogether.*

PER SERVING Calories: 343; Total Fat: 9g; Saturated Fat: 3g; Sodium: 709mg; Carbohydrates: 49g; Fiber: 12g; Protein: 18g

Mushroom and Fennel Stew *over* Egg Noodles

PREP TIME: 10 MINUTES / COOK TIME: 15 MINUTES

Mushrooms and fennel make a beautiful pairing in this satisfying stew. The mushrooms add a deep umami (savory) flavor to the stew, while the fennel adds a subtle anise flavor. Serves 4

2 tablespoons extra-virgin olive oil

1 pound shiitake mushrooms, sliced

1 fennel bulb, trimmed and sliced

2 tablespoons all-purpose flour

1 cup Vegetable Broth (page 184)

2 tablespoons soy sauce

½ cup nonfat sour cream

1 tablespoon Dijon mustard

1 teaspoon dried thyme

¼ cup chopped fresh parsley

2 cups egg noodles, cooked according to package directions

1   In a large skillet, heat the olive oil over medium-high heat until it shimmers.

2   Add the mushrooms and fennel. Cook, stirring occasionally, until the vegetables begin to brown, about 7 minutes.

3   Add the flour and cook, stirring constantly, for 1 minute.

4   Add the vegetable broth and cook, stirring constantly, until it thickens slightly, about 1 minute more.

5   Stir in the soy sauce, sour cream, mustard, and thyme. Cook, stirring constantly, until warmed through, 1 to 2 minutes.

6   Stir in the parsley. Serve warm over the egg noodles.

SUBSTITUTION TIP: *For people with gluten intolerance, replace the flour with a gluten-free flour such as rice flour, and the egg noodles with gluten-free noodles or rice. If you are sensitive to dairy, replace the sour cream with a soy-based sour cream.*

PER SERVING Calories: 313; Total Fat: 10g; Saturated Fat: 2g; Sodium: 1,020mg; Carbohydrates: 50g; Fiber: 6g; Protein: 10g

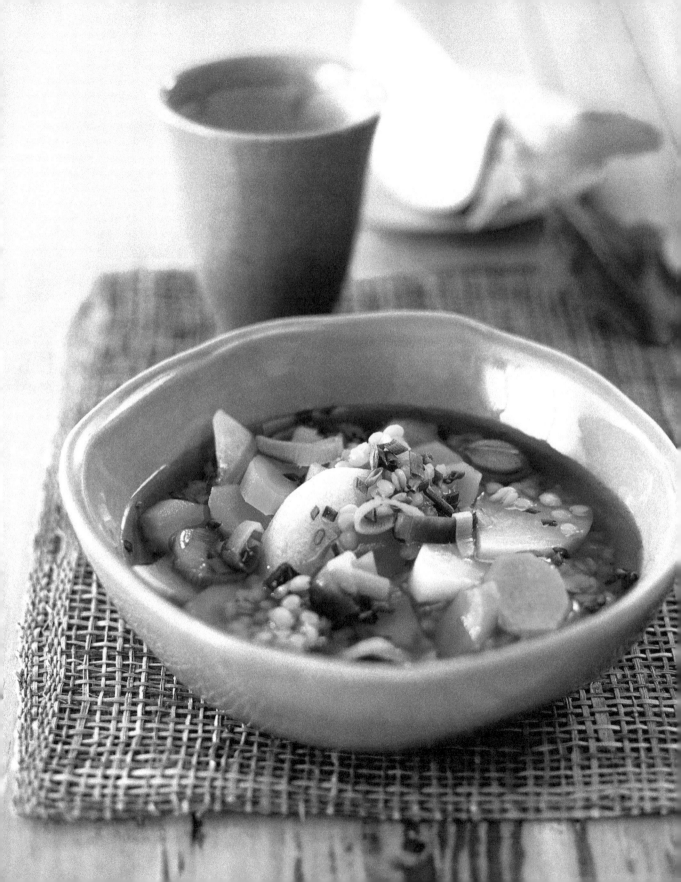

Lentil Vegetable Soup

PREP TIME: 10 MINUTES / COOK TIME: 10 MINUTES

Lentils offer plenty of protein, while a variety of vegetables and herbs make this soup very satisfying. This soup will freeze well for up to 6 months in a tightly sealed container, so it is a great make-ahead meal. Pack it in single-serving containers and take it to work for lunch. Serves 4

2 tablespoons extra-virgin olive oil

2 carrots, peeled and sliced

2 turnips, peeled and sliced

2 okra pods, sliced

1 (14-ounce) can lentils, rinsed and drained

4 cups Vegetable Broth (page 184)

1 teaspoon dried thyme

1 teaspoon salt

1 tablespoon chopped fresh chives (optional)

1   In a large pot, heat the olive oil over medium-high heat until it shimmers.

2   Add the carrots, turnips, and okra and cook, stirring occasionally, until the vegetables are soft, about 6 minutes.

3   Add the lentils, vegetable broth, thyme, and salt. Bring to a simmer and cook for about 4 minutes, until the lentils are heated through.

4   Serve right away, sprinkled with the fresh chives if desired.

SUBSTITUTION TIP: *White beans would also be delicious in this soup. They have a very mild flavor and starchy texture similar to lentils.*

PER SERVING Calories: 496; Total Fat: 10g; Saturated Fat: 2g; Sodium: 1,415mg; Carbohydrates: 71g; Fiber: 34g; Protein: 31g

Roasted Root Vegetable Stew

PREP TIME: 20 MINUTES / COOK TIME: 40 MINUTES

Root vegetables are in season in the fall and the winter, which is the best time to serve this hearty dish. Roasting the vegetables before adding them to the stew adds flavor. Serve it by itself in a bowl, or spoon it over cooked quinoa for an even more satisfying dish. Serves 4

2 sweet potatoes, scrubbed and cut into 1-inch cubes

1 turnip, peeled and cut into 1-inch cubes

1 russet potato, scrubbed and cut into 1-inch cubes

1 large carrot, peeled and cut into 1-inch chunks

2 tablespoons extra-virgin olive oil, divided

1 teaspoon dried thyme

1 teaspoon salt

2 tablespoons all-purpose flour

2 cups Vegetable Broth (page 184)

1 tablespoon Dijon mustard

2 tablespoons chopped fresh parsley

1 Preheat the oven to 450°F.

2 In a large bowl, toss the sweet potatoes, turnip, russet potato, and carrot with 1 tablespoon of olive oil, the dried thyme, and the salt.

3 On two large baking sheets, arrange the vegetables in a single layer. Roast them until they are soft and beginning to brown, about 40 minutes.

4 In a large pot, heat the remaining 1 tablespoon of olive oil over medium-high heat until it shimmers. Add the flour and cook, stirring constantly, for 1 minute.

5 Stir in the vegetable broth and Dijon mustard, cooking until it thickens, about 2 more minutes.

6   Add the roasted root vegetables and stir until they are coated with the vegetable broth mixture.

7   Stir in the parsley and serve.

SUBSTITUTION TIP: *Any root vegetables will work here, with the exception of onions. Feel free to try your own combinations of root veggies to make this tasty stew.*

PER SERVING Calories: 318; Total Fat: 8g; Saturated Fat: 1g; Sodium: 1,055mg; Carbohydrates: 56g; Fiber: 8g; Protein: 7g

Lentil-Carrot Stew

PREP TIME: 10 MINUTES / COOK TIME: 15 MINUTES

Using canned lentils makes this recipe quick and easy, because they cook very quickly. This is a recipe that freezes very well for up to 6 months, so you can make a batch ahead of time to store in your freezer. Serves 6

2 tablespoons extra-virgin olive oil

4 carrots, peeled and cut into ½-inch pieces

1 celery stalk, diced

2 tablespoons all-purpose flour

2 cups Vegetable Broth (page 184)

1 (14-ounce) can lentils, rinsed and drained

1 teaspoon dried tarragon

1 teaspoon salt

1 In a large pot, heat the olive oil over medium-high heat until it shimmers.

2 Add the carrots and celery and cook, stirring occasionally, until soft, about 5 minutes.

3 Add the flour and cook, stirring constantly, for 2 minutes.

4 Add the vegetable broth and cook, stirring constantly, until it thickens, about 2 minutes.

5 Stir in the lentils, tarragon, and salt. Bring to a boil and reduce the heat to medium.

6 Simmer until the carrots are completely soft, about 5 minutes more. Serve warm.

SUBSTITUTION TIP: *If you are gluten intolerant, replace the flour with either rice flour or oat flour.*

PER SERVING Calories: 314; Total Fat: 6g; Saturated Fat: 1g; Sodium: 676mg; Carbohydrates: 46g; Fiber: 21g; Protein: 19g

Quinoa *with* Tofu and Kale

PREP TIME: 10 MINUTES / COOK TIME: 15 MINUTES

Quinoa is packed with protein, while kale is loaded with vitamins and minerals. This makes for a hearty meal that satisfies your hunger while meeting your body's nutritional needs. Serves 4

2½ cups Vegetable Broth, divided (page 184)

1 cup quinoa

1 tablespoon extra-virgin olive oil

1 carrot, peeled and finely chopped

1 tablespoon grated fresh ginger

10 ounces kale, stemmed and torn into bite-size pieces

8 ounces tofu, cut into 1-inch cubes

2 tablespoons soy sauce

Zest of ½ orange, grated

1 tablespoon cornstarch

1   In medium saucepan, combine 2 cups of vegetable broth and the quinoa. Bring to a boil over medium-high heat.

2   Reduce the heat to low and cover the pan. Simmer until the liquid absorbs and the quinoa is tender, 10 to 15 minutes.

3   While the quinoa cooks, heat the olive oil in a large skillet over medium-high heat until it shimmers.

4   Add the carrot and ginger and cook, stirring frequently, until the carrot is soft, about 5 minutes.

5   Add the kale and tofu and cook, stirring frequently, until the kale begins to wilt, about 5 minutes more.

6   In a small bowl, whisk the remaining ½ cup of broth with the soy sauce, orange zest, and cornstarch until well combined. Add the mixture to the skillet and cook until it thickens, about 1 minute

7   Stir in the quinoa and cook for 1 minute more, stirring constantly. Serve warm.

SUBSTITUTION TIP: *If red bell pepper isn't a trigger for you, add ¼ cup minced red pepper with the carrots.*

PER SERVING Calories: 308; Total Fat: 9g; Saturated Fat: 2g; Sodium: 979mg; Carbohydrates: 41g; Fiber: 5g; Protein: 17g

Quinoa Pilau *with* Vegetables

PREP TIME: 15 MINUTES / COOK TIME: 15 MINUTES

This traditional Indian dish has been given a low-acid makeover. Using quinoa in place of rice, the dish is fragrant with delicious herbs and spices. Quinoa is also high in protein, so the meal is very satisfying. Serves 6

2 cups Vegetable Broth (page 184)

1 cup quinoa

2 tablespoons extra-virgin olive oil

1 red bell pepper, seeded and minced

1 cup diced butternut squash

1 tablespoon grated fresh ginger

1 teaspoon salt

½ teaspoon ground cinnamon

½ teaspoon ground cloves

2 tablespoons chopped fresh cilantro

2 tablespoons chopped fresh parsley

2 tablespoons fresh small basil leaves or chopped fresh basil

1   In a medium saucepan, bring the vegetable broth and quinoa to a boil over medium-high heat. Reduce the heat to low, cover, and cook until the liquid absorbs and the quinoa is tender, 10 to 15 minutes.

2   In a large skillet, heat the olive oil over medium-high heat until it shimmers.

3   Add the red pepper, squash, ginger, salt, cinnamon, and cloves. Cook, stirring occasionally, until the vegetables are soft, about 5 minutes.

4   Fluff the quinoa with a fork and add it to the skillet.

5   Stir in the cilantro, parsley, and basil. Serve immediately.

SUBSTITUTION TIP: *This recipe will have a milder, slightly less nutty taste if you use cooked brown rice in place of the quinoa.*

PER SERVING Calories: 268; Total Fat: 11g; Saturated Fat: 2g; Sodium: 970mg; Carbohydrates: 35g; Fiber: 5g; Protein: 9g

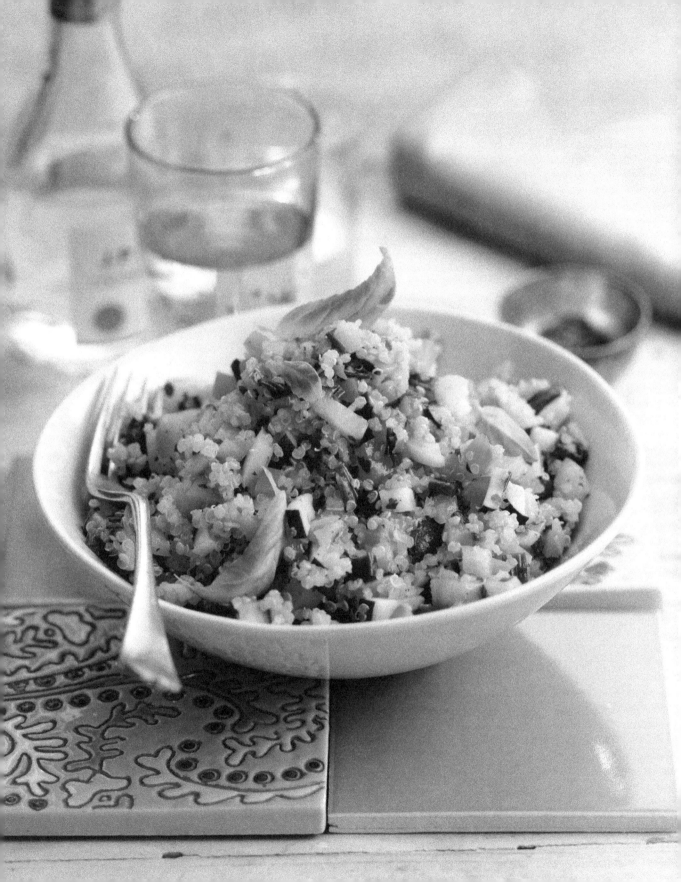

Tofu-Ginger Stir-Fry

**PREP TIME: 15 MINUTES, PLUS 30 MINUTES FOR MARINATING /
COOK TIME: 10 MINUTES**

If you like Asian flavors, then you'll love this stir-fry. Marinating the tofu ahead of time helps the flavors blend into the bean curd, making the entire dish tastier. Finished with lots of veggies, this goes well atop brown rice. Serves 6

¼ cup fresh cilantro leaves and tender stems

Zest of ½ lime, grated

1 teaspoon grated fresh ginger

¼ cup Vegetable Broth (page 184)

2 tablespoons soy sauce

2 tablespoons extra-virgin olive oil, divided

12 ounces firm tofu

1 carrot, peeled and thinly sliced

1 cup broccoli florets

1 cup sliced shiitake mushrooms

1 cup snow peas

1 tablespoon cornstarch

1 tablespoon water

2 cups cooked brown rice

1   In a blender, combine the cilantro, lime zest, ginger, vegetable broth, soy sauce, and 1 tablespoon of olive oil. Blend until smooth.

2   Cut the tofu into 1-inch cubes and put them in a bowl. Add the cilantro-ginger mixture and toss to coat. Set aside to marinate for 30 minutes.

3   In a large skillet, heat the remaining 1 tablespoon of olive oil over medium-high heat until it shimmers.

4   Remove the tofu from the marinade and add it to the pan, reserving the marinade. Add the carrot, broccoli, mushrooms, and peas and cook, stirring frequently, until the vegetables are crisp-tender, about 5 minutes.

5   Add the reserved marinade and bring to a simmer.

6 In a small bowl, whisk together the cornstarch and water. Add this slurry to the skillet and cook, stirring constantly, until the sauce is thick, about 1 minute more.

7 Spoon the mixture over the cooked brown rice and serve.

WHY IT WORKS: *Ginger is great for soothing heartburn, while rice is one of the most calming foods of all. Therefore, this is a great recipe to make if you've been experiencing frequent heartburn recently.*

PER SERVING Calories: 346; Total Fat: 9g; Saturated Fat: 2g; Sodium: 413mg; Carbohydrates: 57g; Fiber: 4g; Protein: 11g

Soba Noodle Salad
with Fava Beans

**PREP TIME: 10 MINUTES, PLUS 2 HOURS FOR CHILLING /
COOK TIME: 10 MINUTES**

Soba noodles are made from buckwheat, and their nutty flavor pairs well with the fava beans and fresh herbs in this salad. For the best marriage of flavors, allow the salad to chill for about 2 hours before serving. Serves 6

4 ounces fava beans

4 ounces soba noodles, cooked according to package directions and cooled

¼ cup extra-virgin olive oil

2 tablespoons soy sauce

1 teaspoon Dijon mustard

½ teaspoon toasted sesame oil

¼ red bell pepper, minced

1 teaspoon grated fresh ginger

¼ cup chopped fresh basil

1   In a saucepan fitted with a steamer basket and lid, steam the fava beans over boiling water for 2 minutes. Rinse under cold water to stop the cooking.

2   Combine the fava beans and cooled soba noodles in a large bowl.

3   In a small bowl, whisk together the olive oil, soy sauce, mustard, sesame oil, red pepper, and ginger.

4   Toss the vinaigrette with the noodles and fava beans. Cover and refrigerate for at least 2 hours.

5   Toss with the fresh basil just before serving.

INGREDIENT SUBSTITUTION: *If you like your noodles with a milder flavor, you can replace the soba noodles with vermicelli or whole-wheat noodles. If you are sensitive to red bell peppers, leave them out of the dish.*

PER SERVING Calories: 314; Total Fat: 14g; Saturated Fat: 2g; Sodium: 694mg; Carbohydrates: 39g; Fiber: 7g; Protein: 12g

Chickpea and Chard Sauté

Made with Mediterranean spices, this chickpea and chard sauté is fragrant and flavorful. It's hearty enough for a winter night's meal, but it also packs well to reheat for a lunch at work. If you'd like a more substantial meal, serve it with brown rice. Serves 4

1 tablespoons extra-virgin olive oil

1 carrot, peeled and diced

1 pound chard, stemmed and torn into bite-size pieces

1 (14-ounce) can chickpeas, rinsed and drained

¼ cup Vegetable Broth (page 184)

2 tablespoons brown sugar

1 teaspoon ground cumin

½ teaspoon ground cinnamon

½ teaspoon salt

1   In a large skillet, heat the olive oil over medium-high heat until it shimmers.

2   Add the carrot and cook, stirring occasionally, until soft, about 5 minutes.

3   Add the chard and cook, stirring occasionally, until soft, about 5 minutes.

4   Stir in the chickpeas, vegetable broth, brown sugar, cumin, cinnamon, and salt. Bring to a boil and reduce the heat to low.

5   Simmer for 5 minutes to allow the flavors to blend. Serve warm.

SUBSTITUTION TIP: *If chard isn't in season, you can replace it with kale or spinach.*

PER SERVING Calories: 442; Total Fat: 10g; Saturated Fat: 1g; Sodium: 617mg; Carbohydrates: 71g; Fiber: 20g; Protein: 22g

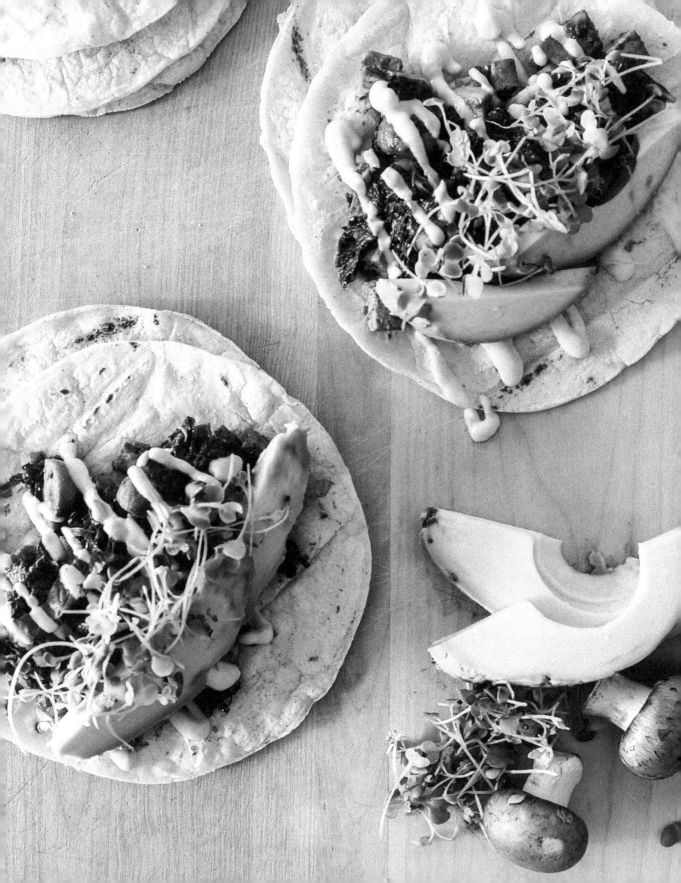

Avocado and Mushroom Tacos

PREP TIME: 15 MINUTES / COOK TIME: 10 MINUTES

Meaty mushrooms sautéed with kale make a tasty filling for corn tortillas. The creamy avocado and cilantro add even more flavor. This is a tasty dinner, and it packs well for lunch the next day, too. Serves 4

8 corn tortillas

2 tablespoons extra-virgin olive oil

6 ounces cremini mushrooms, sliced

1 cup chopped stemmed kale

1 teaspoon grated lime zest

1 teaspoon ground cumin

½ teaspoon salt

1 avocado, peeled, pitted, and sliced

¼ cup chopped fresh cilantro

¼ cup nonfat sour cream

1   Preheat the oven to 350°F.

2   Wrap the corn tortillas in foil and heat them in the oven for 10 minutes.

3   While the tortillas warm, in a large skillet, heat the olive oil over medium-high heat until it shimmers.

4   Add the mushrooms, kale, lime zest, cumin, and salt. Cook, stirring occasionally, until the mushrooms are browned, about 7 minutes.

5   To assemble the tacos, top each tortilla with some of the mushroom mixture, a slice or two of avocado, a sprinkling of cilantro, and a dollop of sour cream. Serve.

INGREDIENT SUBSTITUTION: *Any type of mushrooms will work well in this recipe. Cremini mushrooms, also called baby bellas, have deep, rich flavor that holds up well to the cumin. Button mushrooms aren't as meaty in flavor and take on the flavor of the spices.*

PER SERVING Calories: 304; Total Fat: 18g; Saturated Fat: 3g; Sodium: 339mg; Carbohydrates: 32g; Fiber: 7g; Protein: 6g

Fried Rice

PREP TIME: 10 MINUTES / COOK TIME: 10 MINUTES

This tasty rice is a meal all by itself, or you can serve it as a side for your stir-fry. Fragrant with ginger and filled with crisp-tender pea pods and carrots, this dish is delicious and satisfying without aggravating your acid reflux. Serves 4

1 tablespoons extra-virgin olive oil

1 carrot, peeled and diced

1 cup snow peas

1 tablespoon grated fresh ginger

2 large eggs, beaten

2 cups cooked brown rice

2 tablespoons water

2 tablespoons soy sauce

2 tablespoons chopped fresh cilantro

1   In a large skillet, heat the olive oil over medium-high heat until it shimmers.

2   Add the carrot, peas, and ginger and cook, stirring frequently, until the vegetables are crisp-tender, 4 to 5 minutes.

3   Add the eggs and cook, stirring constantly, until the eggs solidify, about 3 minutes more.

4   Add the rice, water, and soy sauce and cook until warmed through, 2 minutes more.

5   Stir in the cilantro and serve.

INGREDIENT TIP: *To save time, you can purchase precooked brown rice in either the freezer or rice aisle of the grocery store.*

PER SERVING Calories: 428; Total Fat: 8g; Saturated Fat: 2g; Sodium: 521mg; Carbohydrates: 77g; Fiber: 4g; Protein: 11g

Red Beans and Rice

PREP TIME: 10 MINUTES / COOK TIME: 40 MINUTES

Beans and rice combine to make a complete protein, which makes this dish really satisfying. With Southwestern flavors like cilantro and cumin, the meal is also really tasty. Serves 6

2 tablespoons extra-virgin olive oil

1 carrot, peeled and diced

1 celery stalk, peeled and diced

1¾ cups Vegetable Broth (page 184), divided

1 cup brown rice

1 teaspoon ground cumin

1 teaspoon ground coriander

1 teaspoon salt

Zest of ½ lime, grated

1 (14-ounce) can kidney beans, rinsed and drained

¼ cup chopped fresh cilantro

1   In a large saucepan, heat the olive oil over medium-high heat until it shimmers.

2   Add the carrot and celery and cook, stirring occasionally, until the vegetables are soft, about 5 minutes.

3   Add 1½ cups of vegetable broth. Stir in the rice, cumin, coriander, salt, and lime zest.

4   Bring the liquid to a boil. Reduce the heat to medium-low, cover, and simmer for 40 minutes. Then turn off the heat and allow the rice to sit in the covered pot for 10 minutes.

5   Fluff the rice with a fork and return it to medium heat. Stir in the kidney beans and the remaining ¼ cup of stock. Cook, stirring frequently, until the beans are warm, about 5 minutes.

6   Stir in the cilantro and serve.

SUBSTITUTION TIP: *Beyond the initial two weeks of the diet, if you wish you can garnish this dish with 2 tablespoons of grated sharp cheddar cheese.*

PER SERVING Calories: 395; Total Fat: 7g; Saturated Fat: 1g; Sodium: 630mg; Carbohydrates: 66g; Fiber: 12g; Protein: 19g

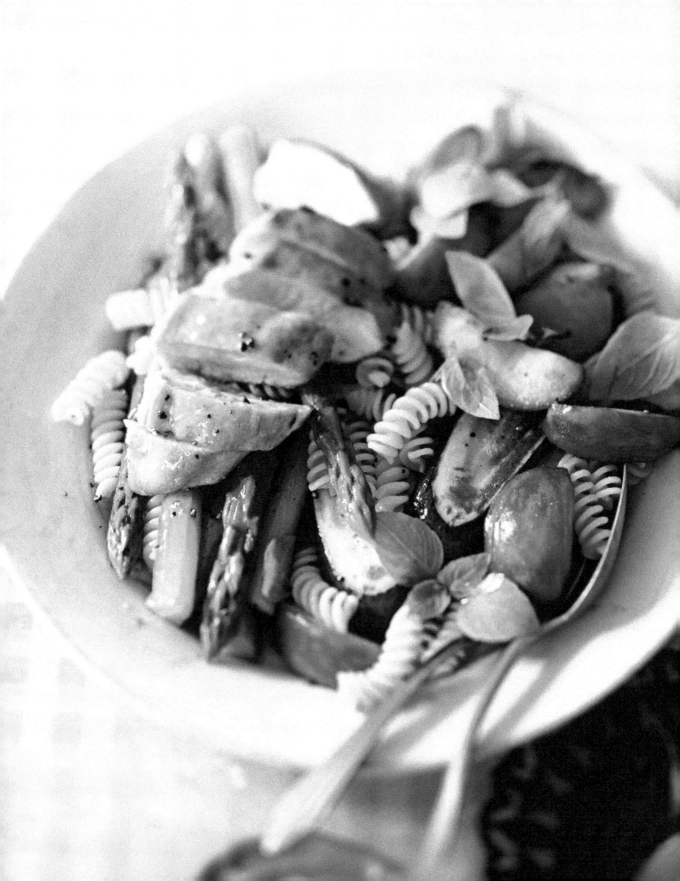

Chapter Eight

Meat and Poultry

Ground Turkey, Mushroom, and Fennel Soup

PREP TIME: 10 MINUTES / COOK TIME: 25 MINUTES

With reflux-soothing fennel, this delicious soup makes a tasty lunch or dinner. It will keep, tightly sealed, for up to 6 months in your freezer. If you're someone who needs a lot of meals on the go, make a double batch. Serves 4

2 tablespoons extra-virgin olive oil, divided

8 ounces ground turkey breast

1 fennel bulb, trimmed and sliced, plus 2 tablespoons chopped fennel fronds

1 large carrot, peeled and cut into 1-inch chunks

8 ounces cremini mushrooms, sliced

5 cups Chicken Broth (page 185)

½ teaspoon salt

1 cup nonfat milk

2 tablespoons cornstarch

1   In a large pot, heat 1 tablespoon of olive oil over medium-high heat until it shimmers.

2   Add the ground turkey and cook, crumbling with a wooden spoon, until browned, about 5 minutes.

3   Remove the turkey with a slotted spoon and transfer to a plate.

4   Heat the remaining 1 tablespoon of olive oil until shimmering. Add the sliced fennel bulb, carrot, and mushrooms and cook, stirring occasionally, until the vegetables begin to brown, 6 to 8 minutes.

5   Stir in the chicken broth, using the side of the spoon to scrape any browned bits from the bottom of the pan. Bring to a simmer and cook until the fennel and carrot are soft, about 5 minutes.

6   Return the turkey to the pot and add the salt.

7   In a small bowl, whisk together the milk and cornstarch until smooth. Pour the mixture into the pot and cook, stirring constantly, until the soup thickens slightly, 3 to 4 minutes.

8   Stir in the chopped fennel fronds and serve.

INGREDIENT TIP: *Not all ground turkey is ground turkey breast. Be sure that the turkey you buy is breast meat (not skin) only. Ground turkey breast will be much lighter in color than ground turkey thighs.*

PER SERVING Calories: 294; Total Fat: 13g; Saturated Fat: 3g; Sodium: 1,359mg; Carbohydrates: 16g; Fiber: 3g; Protein: 27g

Ground Beef and Vegetable Soup

PREP TIME: 10 MINUTES, PLUS 1 TO 2 HOURS FOR MUSHROOMS TO STEEP / COOK TIME: 20 MINUTES

Soaking dried mushrooms in chicken broth and adding a little bit of fish sauce gives this hearty soup a savory, meaty flavor. Dried porcini mushrooms have the most flavor, but any dried mushrooms will work. You can use any vegetables you like in this soup (with the exception of green peppers and cucumbers), so feel free to experiment. Serves 4

5 cups Chicken Broth (page 185)

2 ounces dried mushrooms

2 tablespoons extra-virgin olive oil, divided

8 ounces extra-lean ground beef

2 carrots, peeled and chopped

2 celery stalks, chopped

1 zucchini, chopped

1 sweet potato, peeled and chopped

4 ounces green beans, chopped

2 teaspoons fish sauce

1 teaspoon dried thyme

½ teaspoon salt

1   In a medium saucepan, bring the chicken broth to a simmer over medium heat.

2   Remove the pan from the heat and add the dried mushrooms.

3   Cover the pan and allow the mushrooms to steep for 1 to 2 hours.

4   In a large pot, heat 1 tablespoon of olive oil over medium-high heat until it shimmers.

5   Add the ground beef and cook, crumbling with a wooden spoon, until browned, about 5 minutes. Remove the beef with a slotted spoon and transfer it to a plate.

6   Heat the remaining 1 tablespoon of oil until it shimmers.

7   Add the carrots and celery and cook, stirring occasionally, until the vegetables begin to brown, 5 to 7 minutes.

8   When the soaked mushrooms are soft, remove them from the broth (reserve the broth) and chop. Add the broth and the soaked mushrooms, scraping any browned bits from the bottom of the pot with the side of the spoon.

9   Stir in the zucchini, sweet potato, green beans, fish sauce, thyme, and salt. Bring the mixture to a simmer. Reduce the heat to medium and allow the soup to simmer until the vegetables are tender, about 5 minutes.

10 Return the ground beef to the pan. Simmer for another minute or two, until the beef is heated through. Serve warm.

INGREDIENT TIP: *When ground beef lists its fat percentage, it labels it by volume and not by calories. Extra-lean ground beef has 95 or 96 percent by volume lean beef and 4 to 5 percent fat. If you can't find extra-lean beef, substitute ground turkey breast instead.*

PER SERVING Calories: 289; Total Fat: 11g; Saturated Fat: 3g; Sodium: 1,556mg; Carbohydrates: 21g; Fiber: 7g; Protein: 24g

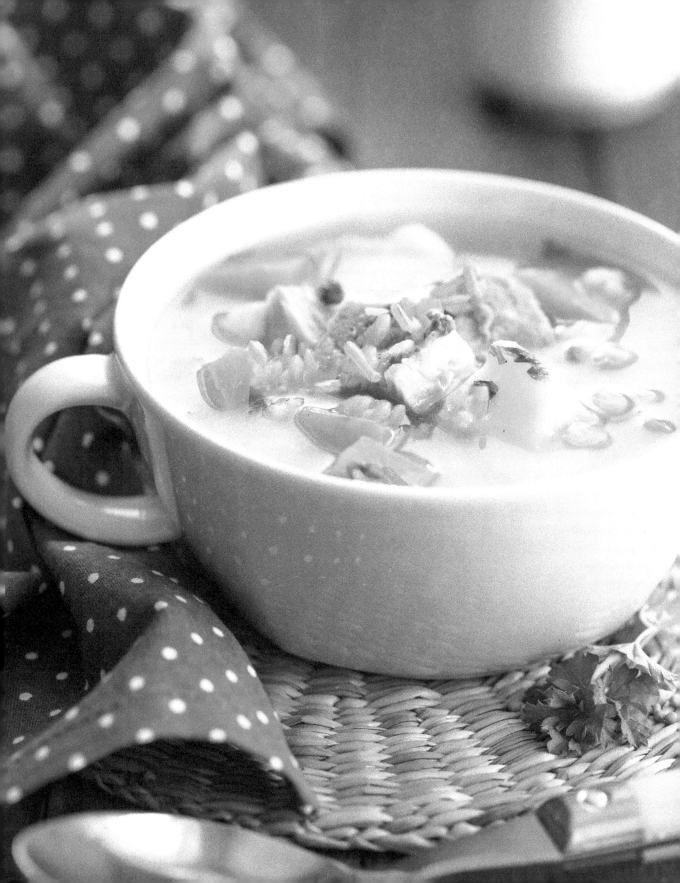

Ginger Chicken and Rice Soup

PREP TIME: 10 MINUTES / COOK TIME: 20 MINUTES

This warming soup is not only satisfying, but it is fragrant with one of the best ingredients for acid reflux: ginger. With a savory Asian flavor profile and hearty chicken, vegetables, and brown rice, this tasty soup will tickle your taste buds without aggravating your reflux. Serves 4

2 tablespoons extra-virgin olive oil, divided

8 ounces boneless, skinless chicken breast, cut into ½-inch pieces

2 carrots, peeled and chopped

2 celery stalks, chopped

1 tablespoon grated fresh ginger

5 cups Chicken Broth (page 185)

2 teaspoons fish sauce

1 cup peas (fresh or frozen)

1 cup hot, cooked brown rice

1   In a large pot, heat 1 tablespoon of olive oil over medium-high heat until it shimmers.

2   Add the chicken and cook, stirring occasionally, until cooked through, 5 to 7 minutes.

3   Remove the chicken with a slotted spoon and transfer it to a plate.

4   Heat the remaining 1 tablespoon of oil until it shimmers.

5   Add the carrots, celery, and ginger. Cook, stirring occasionally, until the vegetables begin to brown, 5 to 7 minutes.

6   Add the chicken broth and fish sauce, scraping any browned bits from the bottom of the pan with the side of the spoon.

7   Stir in the peas and mushrooms. Bring to a simmer and then reduce the heat to medium-low. Simmer until the peas are cooked, 3 to 4 minutes.

8   Divided the cooked brown rice among four bowls. Ladle the soup over the top and serve.

PER SERVING Calories: 422; Total Fat: 12g; Saturated Fat: 2g; Sodium: 1,283mg; Carbohydrates: 47g; Fiber: 5g; Protein: 30g

Beef and Vegetable Stir-Fry *with* Basil

PREP TIME: 15 MINUTES / COOK TIME: 10 MINUTES

Cutting the beef into very thin slices makes this stir-fry come together quickly. Serve it by itself, or include a small serving of rice to soak up the juices. Adding fresh basil at the end provides a nice, peppery bite to the dish. Serves 4

2 tablespoons extra-virgin olive oil

1 teaspoon toasted sesame oil

1 (12-ounce) flank steak, thinly sliced against the grain

2 carrots, peeled and sliced

2 celery stalks, sliced

1 tablespoon grated fresh ginger

2 tablespoons soy sauce

¼ cup small fresh basil leaves or chopped fresh basil

1   In a large skillet, heat the olive oil and sesame oil over medium-high heat until it shimmers.

2   Add the steak slices and cook, stirring occasionally, until they are cooked through, about 4 minutes. Use tongs to transfer the steak to a plate.

3   Add the carrots, celery, and ginger to the skillet and cook, stirring occasionally, until the vegetables are browned, about 5 minutes.

4   Return the steak to the pan and stir in the soy sauce. Cook until the steak rewarms, about 2 minutes.

5   Stir in the fresh basil just before serving.

   COOKING TIP: *To make it easy to cut thin slices from the flank steak, freeze it for 30 minutes just before slicing, and use a very sharp knife.*

   PER SERVING Calories: 258; Total Fat: 15g; Saturated Fat: 4g; Sodium: 527mg; Carbohydrates: 5g; Fiber: 1g; Protein: 24g

Spaghetti *with* Ground Turkey and Broccolini

PREP TIME: 10 MINUTES / COOK TIME: 15 MINUTES

Ginger marries well with broccolini in this sweet and savory stir-fry that tops spaghetti. Choose whole-wheat spaghetti for extra fiber. Serves 4

2 tablespoons extra-virgin olive oil, divided

8 ounces ground turkey breast

8 ounces broccolini, trimmed

2 tablespoons grated fresh ginger

¼ cup Chicken Broth (page 185)

2 tablespoons soy sauce

2 tablespoons cornstarch

2 tablespoons brown sugar

4 ounces spaghetti, cooked according to package directions

¼ cup chopped fresh cilantro

1 In a large skillet, heat 1 tablespoon of olive oil over medium-high heat until it shimmers.

2 Add the ground turkey and cook, crumbling with a wooden spoon, until it is browned, about 5 minutes.

3 Remove the turkey with a slotted spoon and transfer it to a plate.

4 Heat the remaining 1 tablespoon of olive oil until it shimmers.

5 Add the broccolini and ginger and cook, stirring occasionally, until the broccolini is crisp-tender, about 5 minutes.

6 In a small bowl, whisk together the chicken broth, soy sauce, cornstarch, and brown sugar until smooth. Add the mixture to the skillet, along with the reserved ground turkey.

7 Cook, stirring constantly, for 1 minute longer.

8 Toss the sauce with the spaghetti and cilantro and serve.

SUBSTITUTION TIP: *If you can't find broccolini, replace it with broccoli florets that have been cut into very small pieces.*

PER SERVING Calories: 321; Total Fat: 12g; Saturated Fat: 2g; Sodium: 561mg; Carbohydrates: 30g; Fiber: 1g; Protein: 23g

Turkey Breast Cutlets *with* Mashed Potatoes and Mushroom Gravy

PREP TIME: 10 MINUTES / COOK TIME: 20 MINUTES

If you're a Thanksgiving dinner fan, then you'll love this quick turkey breast dinner. Using thin-sliced turkey cutlets allows you to cook the turkey quickly on your stovetop. The pan drippings make for a savory gravy. Serves 4

2 tablespoons extra-virgin olive oil, divided

1 pound turkey breast cutlets

1 teaspoon salt, divided

4 ounces cremini mushrooms, sliced

1 teaspoon dried rosemary

1 teaspoon dried thyme

2 cups Chicken Broth (page 185)

2 tablespoons cornstarch

2 tablespoons water

1 teaspoon fish sauce

1 recipe Loaded Mashed Potatoes (page 102), made without the turkey bacon

1   In a large skillet, heat 1 tablespoon of olive oil over medium-high heat until it shimmers.

2   Sprinkle the turkey cutlets with ½ teaspoon of salt.

3   Add the turkey cutlets to the hot oil and cook until cooked through, 2 to 3 minutes per side. Transfer the cutlets to a plate.

4   Heat the remaining 1 tablespoon of olive oil until it shimmers.

5   Add the mushrooms, rosemary, thyme, and remaining ½ teaspoon of salt. Cook, stirring occasionally, until the mushrooms are deeply browned, 7 to 8 minutes.

6   Add the chicken broth, scraping any browned bits from the bottom of the pan with the side of a wooden spoon. Bring to a simmer.

7   In a small bowl, whisk together the cornstarch, water, and fish sauce. Add the mixture to the skillet and cook, stirring constantly, until the gravy thickens, 1 to 2 minutes more.

8   Serve the turkey cutlets and potatoes topped with the gravy.

SUBSTITUTION TIP: *If you can't find turkey cutlets, you can make your own from a skinless turkey breast. Slice the breast crosswise into ½-inch slices and then pound the meat slightly to even out the thickness.*

PER SERVING Calories: 365; Total Fat: 15g; Saturated Fat: 5g; Sodium: 1,589mg; Carbohydrates: 24g; Fiber: 3g; Protein: 35g

Chicken Legs with Potatoes

PREP TIME: 10 MINUTES / COOK TIME: 50 MINUTES

Chicken hindquarters have a little more fat than chicken breasts, particularly with the skin on. If fat really triggers your GERD, then remove the skin before roasting the chicken. You can use any type of potatoes in this recipe if you can't find fingerlings. Serves 4

4 chicken legs (thigh and drumstick pieces together)

8 fingerling potatoes, quartered

4 large carrots, peeled and cut into sticks

1 tablespoon extra-virgin olive oil

1 teaspoon dried thyme

1 teaspoon salt

1 tablespoon chopped fresh chives

1 Preheat the oven to 425°F.

2 In a large baking dish or roasting pan, toss the chicken, potatoes, and carrots with the olive oil, thyme, and salt.

3 Bake until the chicken juices run clear, about 50 minutes.

4 Sprinkle with the chives before serving.

SUBSTITUTION TIP: *To cut back on fat, try this recipe with boneless, skinless chicken breasts.*

PER SERVING Calories: 579; Total Fat: 20g; Saturated Fat: 5g; Sodium: 877mg; Carbohydrates: 75g; Fiber: 9g; Protein: 28g

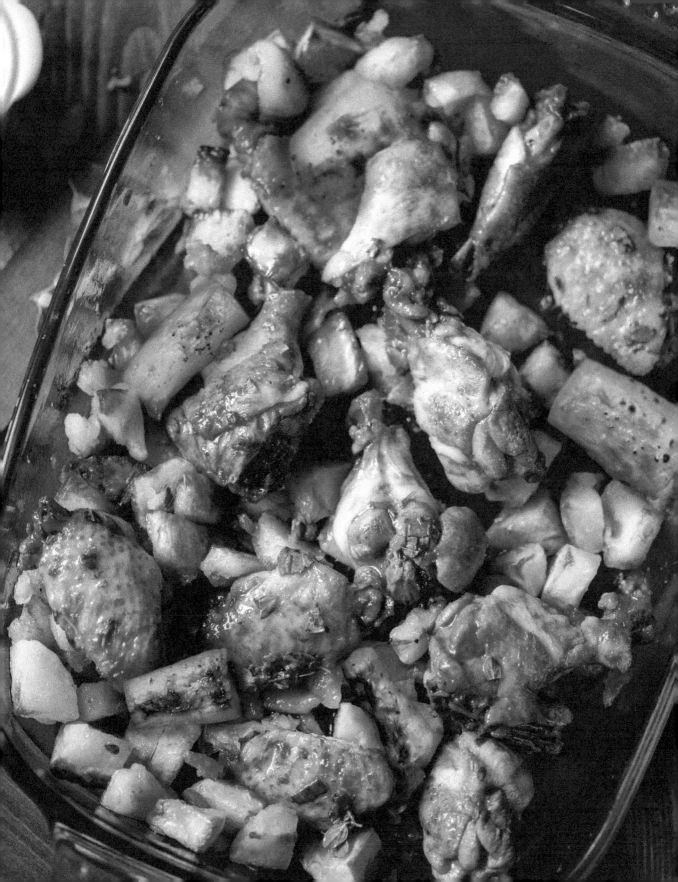

Savory Turkey Burgers

PREP TIME: 10 MINUTES / COOK TIME: 10 MINUTES

Adding fish sauce, salt, and sugar lends a meaty, savory flavor to these turkey burgers. Serve them alongside Baked Sweet Potato Chips (page 89), or with a side of baby carrots. If you make these for a work lunch, cook the patties and then bring the buns and sauce separately, assembling the burgers right before you eat. Serves 4

1 pound ground turkey breast

1 tablespoon fish sauce

1 tablespoon brown sugar

1 teaspoon ground cumin

¼ teaspoon salt

1 tablespoon extra-virgin olive oil

4 whole-wheat hamburger buns

4 tablespoons Mediterranean Chickpea Spread (page 195)

2 ounces arugula

1   In a medium bowl, mix the ground turkey breast, fish sauce, brown sugar, cumin, and salt until well combined.

2   Form the mixture into four patties.

3   In a large skillet, heat the olive oil over medium-high heat until it shimmers.

4   Add the turkey patties and cook until cooked through, about 5 minutes per side.

5   Spread each bun bottom with 1 tablespoon of chickpea spread. Add the turkey burger and top with the arugula. Serve.

SUBSTITUTION TIP: *Beyond the initial two weeks of the diet, if you find you can tolerate a small amount of cheese, add 2 tablespoons of crumbled feta to each burger before serving.*

PER SERVING Calories: 379; Total Fat: 15g; Saturated Fat: 5g; Sodium: 753mg; Carbohydrates: 24g; Fiber: 4g; Protein: 38g

Baked Chicken Tenders

PREP TIME: 15 MINUTES / COOK TIME: 15 MINUTES

If you love fried chicken, with its crunchy coating, then these chicken tenders can help satisfy that craving. Coat them in panko bread crumbs, which bake up extra crispy. Serve them with a simple salad, or alongside Smoky Baked Beans (page 101), with Orange-Honey-Dijon Dressing (page 187) as a dipping sauce. Serves 4

1 cup panko bread crumbs

½ teaspoon dried thyme

½ teaspoon salt

2 large eggs, beaten

½ cup nonfat buttermilk

1 teaspoon Dijon mustard

½ cup all-purpose flour

1 pound boneless, skinless chicken breast, cut into ½-inch-thick strips

1   Preheat the oven to 375°F.

2   Line a baking sheet with parchment paper or aluminum foil.

3   In a shallow dish or pie plate, mix the bread crumbs, thyme, and salt.

4   In another shallow dish, whisk together the eggs, buttermilk, and Dijon mustard.

5   Put the flour in a third shallow dish.

6   Dredge each chicken strip in the flour, coating it. Tap off any excess flour.

7   Dip each strip into the egg mixture, and then into the bread crumb mixture, coating it completely.

8   Lay the chicken strips on the lined baking sheet and bake until cooked through, about 15 minutes. Serve warm.

INGREDIENT TIP: *If you can't find panko, use any type of prepared bread crumbs, or make your own from stale bread pulsed in a food processor until crumbly.*

PER SERVING Calories: 358; Total Fat: 7g; Saturated Fat: 1g; Sodium: 636mg; Carbohydrates: 29g; Fiber: 3g; Protein: 44g

Chicken, Pasta, Asparagus, and Red Potato Salad

**PREP TIME: 15 MINUTES, PLUS 30 MINUTES FOR CHILLING /
COOK TIME: 20 MINUTES**

Roasting the vegetables gives this chicken salad a depth of flavor you wouldn't get using steamed vegetables. Most supermarkets offer cooked chicken breast at the salad bar or in the deli area where they sell rotisserie chicken. Be sure to remove the skin before slicing the breast. Alternatively, you can simply grill a chicken breast for about 7 minutes per side. Serves 6

4 baby red potatoes, quartered

4 ounces asparagus, trimmed

1 zucchini, sliced

6 tablespoons extra-virgin olive oil, divided

1 cup rotini pasta, cooked and cooled

12 ounces boneless, skinless chicken breast, cooked and sliced

2 tablespoons apple cider vinegar

1 teaspoon Dijon mustard

1 teaspoon salt

¼ cup small fresh basil leaves or chopped fresh basil

1 Preheat the oven to 450°F.

2 In a large bowl, toss the potatoes, asparagus, and zucchini with 2 tablespoons of olive oil.

3 Arrange the vegetables in a single layer on a large baking sheet. Roast until the potatoes are tender, about 20 minutes. Allow to cool completely.

4 In a large bowl, combine the potato mixture, pasta, and chicken.

5 In a small bowl, whisk together the vinegar, mustard, salt, and the remaining 4 tablespoons of olive oil.

6   Toss the dressing with the salad. Cover and refrigerate for about 30 minutes to allow the flavors to blend.

7   Stir in the basil just before serving.

INGREDIENT TIP: *Add ¼ cup Parmesan cheese just before serving to lend a richer flavor to the salad.*

PER SERVING Calories: 359; Total Fat: 7g; Saturated Fat: 17g; Sodium: 472mg; Carbohydrates: 31g; Fiber: 2g; Protein: 24g

Orange-Ginger Chicken Stir-Fry

PREP TIME: 15 MINUTES / COOK TIME: 20 MINUTES

Orange zest and ginger blend beautifully in this quick and easy stir-fry, offering a sweet, slightly zippy, and flavorful topping for cooked brown rice. This is a recipe that customizes well, allowing you to add any vegetables you wish. Serves 4

2 tablespoons extra-virgin olive oil, divided

8 ounces boneless, skinless chicken breast, cut into 1-inch pieces

½ teaspoon toasted sesame oil

1 cup sugar snap peas

1 carrot, peeled and thinly sliced

4 ounces canned water chestnuts, drained and sliced

2 tablespoons grated fresh ginger

¼ cup Chicken Broth (page 185)

2 tablespoons soy sauce

2 tablespoons honey

1 tablespoon cornstarch

Zest of 1 orange, grated

1 cup cooked brown rice

1   In a large skillet, heat 1 tablespoon of olive oil over medium-high heat until it shimmers.

2   Add the chicken and cook, stirring occasionally, until browned, 5 to 7 minutes.

3   Remove the chicken from the skillet with tongs and transfer to a plate.

4   Heat the remaining 1 tablespoon of olive oil and the sesame oil until it shimmers.

5   Add the pea pods, carrot, water chestnuts, and ginger. Cook, stirring occasionally, until the vegetables are tender, 5 to 7 minutes.

6   In a small bowl, whisk together the chicken broth, soy sauce, honey, cornstarch, and orange zest. Add the mixture to the skillet, along with the reserved chicken.

7 Bring to a simmer and cook, stirring constantly, until the sauce thickens slightly, about 2 minutes.

8 Serve the stir-fry over the rice.

INGREDIENT TIP: *When zesting citrus peel, make sure you don't get any of the white part just under the zest, called the pith. The pith is bitter and will impart unpleasant flavors to your food. Use a rasp-style grater for best results when zesting.*

PER SERVING Calories: 442; Total Fat: 11g; Saturated Fat: 1g; Sodium: 582mg; Carbohydrates: 61g; Fiber: 3g; Protein: 24g

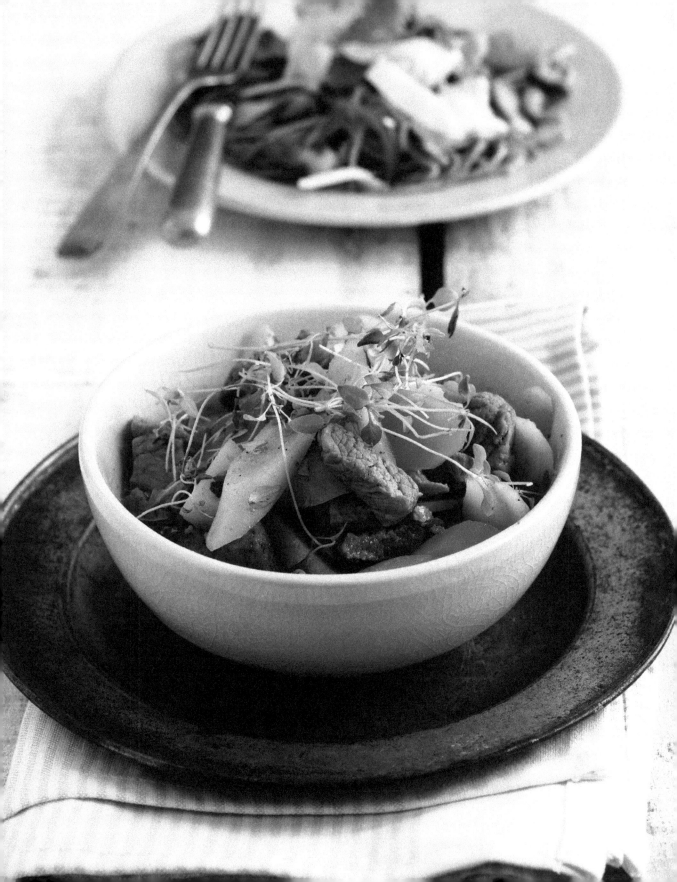

Steak Salad *with* Root Vegetables and Watercress

PREP TIME: 20 MINUTES, PLUS COOLING TIME / COOK TIME: 45 MINUTES

This dish is served cold, making it an excellent choice for lunch to take to work. Just keep it in an airtight container in your fridge for up to 5 days for a hearty yet tasty meal. Serves 6

3 large carrots, peeled and cut into 1-inch chunks

2 turnips, peeled and cut into 1-inch chunks

2 parsnips, peeled and cut into 1-inch chunks

6 tablespoons extra-virgin olive oil, divided

1 teaspoon salt, divided

1 (12-ounce) flank steak

2 cups watercress, plus more for optional garnish

2 tablespoons red wine vinegar

2 tablespoons soy sauce

1 tablespoon Dijon mustard

1 tablespoon chopped fresh thyme

1 Preheat the oven to 425°F.

2 Toss the carrots, turnips, and parsnips with 2 tablespoons of olive oil and ½ teaspoon of salt, and spread them in a single layer on two baking sheets.

3 Roast until the vegetables begin to brown, about 45 minutes. Set aside the vegetables to cool completely.

4 While the vegetables are roasting, season the flank steak with the remaining ½ teaspoon of salt.

5 In a large skillet, heat 1 tablespoon of oil over medium-high heat until it shimmers.

6 Add the flank steak and cook for about 5 minutes per side for medium-rare. Transfer the steak to a cutting board and allow it to cool completely. ▸

7   When the steak is cooled, cut it against the grain into ½-inch-thick slices.

8   Transfer the steak slices to a large bowl, along with the cooled vegetables and the watercress.

9   In a small bowl, whisk the remaining 3 tablespoons of olive oil with the vinegar, soy sauce, mustard, and thyme.

10 Toss the vinaigrette with the salad and serve cold, garnished with additional watercress if desired.

COOKING TIP: *Tri-tip and sirloin steak also work well in this recipe. Tri-tip has an especially rich flavor.*

PER SERVING Calories: 300; Total Fat: 19g; Saturated Fat: 4g; Sodium: 813mg; Carbohydrates: 15g; Fiber: 4g; Protein: 18g

Hamburger Stroganoff

PREP TIME: 10 MINUTES / COOK TIME: 20 MINUTES

Stroganoff is a traditional Russian dish, typically made with strips of tender beef. Using extra-lean ground beef here lowers the fat and makes the preparation a lot easier. Serves 4

1 pound extra-lean ground beef

2 tablespoons extra-virgin olive oil

8 ounces cremini mushrooms, sliced

1 teaspoon dried thyme

½ teaspoon salt

2 cups Chicken Broth (page 185)

1 tablespoon Dijon mustard

1 teaspoon fish sauce

1 tablespoon brown sugar

1 tablespoon cornstarch

½ cup nonfat sour cream

¼ cup chopped fresh parsley

2 cups egg noodles, cooked according to package directions

1   Heat a large skillet over medium-high heat. Add the ground beef and cook, crumbling with a wooden spoon, until browned, about 5 minutes. Using a slotted spoon, remove the beef from the skillet and set it aside.

2   In the same skillet, heat the olive oil until it shimmers. Add the mushrooms, thyme, and salt and cook, stirring occasionally, until well browned, 6 to 8 minutes.

3   In a bowl, whisk together the chicken broth, mustard, fish sauce, brown sugar, and cornstarch until blended. Add the mixture to the mushrooms in the pan, along with the reserved ground beef.

4   Cook, stirring constantly, until the beef heats through and the sauce thickens slightly, about 3 minutes.

5   Stir in the sour cream and cook, stirring constantly, until warm, 1 or 2 minutes more.

6   Stir in the parsley and serve spooned over the egg noodles.

PER SERVING Calories: 397; Total Fat: 14g; Saturated Fat: 4g; Sodium: 938mg; Carbohydrates: 33g; Fiber: 2g; Protein: 33g

Asparagus, Spinach, and Chicken Roulade

PREP TIME: 20 MINUTES / COOK TIME: 35 MINUTES

A roulade is merely one thing rolled around another. For example, in baking, a jellyroll is a roulade. With this dish, chicken breast is rolled around asparagus and spinach, making a delicious all-in-one meal. Serves 4

1 pound boneless, skinless chicken breast

1 teaspoon salt, divided

1 tablespoon extra-virgin olive oil

10 ounces baby spinach

Zest of ½ orange, grated

8 ounces asparagus spears, trimmed

1   Preheat the oven to 425°F.

2   Line a baking sheet with parchment paper or aluminum foil. Place four wooden skewers or toothpicks in a dish of water to soak.

3   Cut the chicken breast horizontally into four equal-size filets. Put each filet between two sheets of parchment paper or plastic wrap and pound to a ¼-inch thickness.

4   Season each chicken piece with ⅛ teaspoon of salt.

5   In a large skillet, heat the olive oil over medium-high heat until it shimmers. Add the baby spinach, the remaining ½ teaspoon of salt, and the orange zest. Cook, stirring constantly, until the spinach wilts, about 2 minutes.

6   Remove the skillet from the heat and set aside to cool for 5 minutes.

7   Spread an equal amount of the spinach mixture evenly over each pounded chicken breast filet. Top each with two or three asparagus spears.

8   Roll the chicken around the filling and insert a wooden skewer or toothpick to hold the roll together.

9   Place the chicken rolls on the lined baking sheet and bake until the juices run clear, about 30 minutes. Serve warm.

COOKING TIP: *Soaking the wooden skewers or toothpicks in water for 30 minutes will keep them from smoking or burning in the hot oven.*

PER SERVING Calories: 244; Total Fat: 8g; Saturated Fat: 1g; Sodium: 769mg; Carbohydrates: 5g; Fiber: 3g; Protein: 40g

Pork Tenderloin *with* Apples and Fennel

PREP TIME: 15 MINUTES / COOK TIME: 40 MINUTES

This tasty dinner is as simple as searing the seasoned tenderloin and then roasting it with the apples and fennel. You'll have dinner on the table in less than an hour, with very little hands-on work time, making it perfect for a busy weekday night. Cooking it in an oven-proof pan, such as a cast iron skillet, also makes cleanup easy because you need only one pot. Serves 4

1 pound pork tenderloin

1 teaspoon salt

1 teaspoon dried thyme

½ teaspoon sage

1 tablespoon extra-virgin olive oil

2 red apples, such as Fuji, peeled, cored, and sliced

1 fennel bulb, trimmed and thinly sliced

1 tablespoon Dijon mustard

1 cup Chicken Broth (page 185)

1 tablespoon brown sugar

1   Preheat the oven to 425°F.

2   Rub the pork all over with the salt, thyme, and sage.

3   In a large, ovenproof skillet, heat the olive oil over medium-high heat until it shimmers.

4   Add the pork to the hot oil and cook until it is well browned on all sides, 12 to 15 minutes total.

5   Transfer the pork to a platter.

6   Add the apples and fennel to the skillet and cook, stirring occasion-ally, until the apples begin to brown, about 5 minutes.

7   Brush the pork with the mustard and return it to the pan.

8   Roast in the oven until the pork reaches an internal temperature of 145°F on an instant-read thermometer, 10 to 15 minutes.

9   Transfer the pork to a platter, tent it with foil, and let it rest for
    10 minutes.

10 While the pork rests, set the skillet with the apples and fennel on the
    stovetop over medium-high heat.

11 Stir in the chicken broth, scraping any browned bits from the bottom
    of the pan with the side of a wooden spoon.

12 Stir in the brown sugar. Simmer for 5 minutes.

13 Slice the pork loin and serve with the apple-fennel mixture spooned
    over the top.

COOKING TIP: *Adding the chicken stock and scraping the browned bits from the bottom of the pan, a step called deglazing, is important in this and many recipes. When you cook meat and vegetables, they caramelize on the surface, leaving little bits of flavor in the pan. Adding liquid and scraping them up with a spoon allows you to gather all those little pieces of deliciousness and incorporate them into your dish.*

PER SERVING Calories: 232; Total Fat: 5g; Saturated Fat: 2g; Sodium: 912mg; Carbohydrates: 15g; Fiber: 4g; Protein: 32g

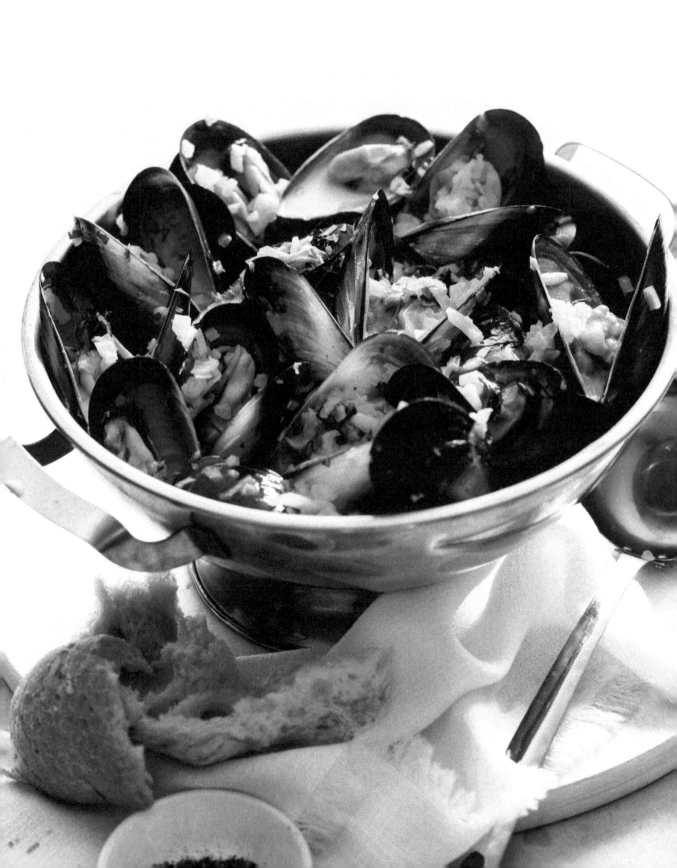

Fish and Shellfish

New England Clam Chowder

PREP TIME: 10 MINUTES / COOK TIME: 25 MINUTES

New England clam chowder is a favorite for many, but it's a nightmare for heartburn sufferers. With lots of fat, as well as onions, it can cause acid reflux. This version is lower in fat and substitutes soothing fennel for the heartburn-causing ingredients. Serves 4

1 tablespoon extra-virgin olive oil

2 ounces turkey bacon, cut into pieces

1 fennel bulb, trimmed and chopped, plus 2 tablespoons chopped fennel fronds

2 large carrots, peeled and chopped

4 cups Chicken Broth (page 185)

1 cup clam juice

1 teaspoon salt

8 ounces clam meat (canned or fresh)

1 russet potato, peeled and chopped

¼ cup corn (frozen, canned, or fresh)

1 cup nonfat milk

2 tablespoons cornstarch

1   In a large pot, heat the olive oil over medium-high heat until it shimmers.

2   Add the turkey bacon and cook, stirring occasionally, until browned, about 5 minutes.

3   Add the chopped fennel bulb and carrots and cook, stirring occasionally, until the vegetables begin to brown slightly, about 5 minutes more.

4   Add the chicken broth, clam juice, and salt, using the side of a wooden spoon to scrape any browned bits from the bottom of the pan.

5   Add the clams, potatoes, and corn. Cook, stirring occasionally, until the potatoes are tender, about 10 minutes.

6   In a small bowl, whisk together the milk and cornstarch. Add the mixture to the pot and cook, stirring constantly, until the soup thickens slightly, about 2 minutes.

7   Stir in the fennel fronds and serve.

INGREDIENT TIP: *When you buy whole fennel, it comes with a bulb, stalks, and fronds. The fronds make wonderful seasoning, adding a fresh flavor when added at the end of the recipe. Save any trimmings in a resealable bag in the freezer to use making vegetable or chicken broth.*

PER SERVING Calories: 323; Total Fat: 7g; Saturated Fat: 1g; Sodium: 1,827mg; Carbohydrates: 36g; Fiber: 4g; Protein: 27g

Steamer Clams *with* Lemon and Fennel

PREP TIME: 10 MINUTES / COOK TIME: 15 MINUTES

Steamer clams cook quickly and make a delicious meal or appetizer. They are best when really fresh, so don't plan on saving leftovers. In this version, fennel adds a delicate anise flavor to the sweet clams. Serve with crusty bread to dip in the clam nectar. Serves 4

1 tablespoon extra-virgin olive oil

1 fennel bulb, trimmed and chopped, plus 2 tablespoons chopped fennel fronds

4 pounds fresh steamer clams in their shells, cleaned

3 cups Chicken Broth (page 185)

Zest of 1 lemon, grated

½ teaspoon salt

1   In a large pot, heat the olive oil over medium-high heat until it shimmers.

2   Add the chopped fennel bulb and cook, stirring occasionally, until slightly brown, about 5 minutes.

3   Add the clams, chicken broth, lemon zest, and salt. Cover and cook until the clams open, 7 to 10 minutes.

4   Stir in the fennel fronds. Ladle into bowls and serve.

INGREDIENT TIP: *Discard any clams that don't open after steaming, as they are dead, and may contain bacteria or toxins.*

PER SERVING Calories: 467; Total Fat: 15g; Saturated Fat: 3g; Sodium: 1,410mg; Carbohydrates: 22g; Fiber: 2g; Protein: 58g

Mussels in Broth *with* Tarragon

PREP TIME: 10 MINUTES / COOK TIME: 15 MINUTES

Mussels steam quickly, making for a quick meal. Be sure to discard any mussels that don't open after steaming. Tarragon adds a delicate anise-like flavor to these delicious mussels. Instead of serving these mussels with rice, you can sop up the broth with crusty bread. Serves 4

3 cups Chicken Broth (page 185)

Zest of 1 orange, grated

2 tablespoons dried tarragon

½ teaspoon salt

4 pounds mussels, cleaned and debearded

1 cup cooked brown rice

2 tablespoons chopped fresh parsley

¼ cup grated Parmesan cheese (optional)

1   In a large pot, combine the chicken broth, orange zest, tarragon, and salt. Add the mussels.

2   Bring to a boil over medium-high heat, cover the pot, and cook until the mussels open, 5 to 10 minutes.

3   Stir in the rice and parsley.

4   Sprinkle with the Parmesan cheese (if using) and serve in shallow bowls.

INGREDIENT TIP: *To debeard mussels, use a very sharp paring knife to carefully cut the stringy beard away from the shell.*

PER SERVING Calories: 344; Total Fat: 7g; Saturated Fat: 3g; Sodium: 1,323mg; Carbohydrates: 43g; Fiber: 1g; Protein: 25g

Brazilian Fish Stew

PREP TIME: 10 MINUTES / COOK TIME: 30 MINUTES

This fish stew borrows its flavors from a Brazilian dish called *moqueca*. With plenty of lime, cumin, and cilantro, it's a tasty way to enjoy fish. While this recipe calls for cod, you can replace it with any white fish. Serves 4

1 tablespoon extra-virgin olive oil

2 large carrots, peeled and chopped

1 cup Chicken Broth (page 185)

1 cup light coconut milk

Zest of 1 lime, grated

2 teaspoons ground cumin

½ teaspoon salt

8 ounces red baby potatoes, quartered

1 pound cod fillets, cut into 1-inch pieces

2 tablespoons cornstarch

2 tablespoons water

¼ cup chopped fresh cilantro

1   In a large pot, heat the olive oil over medium-high heat until it shimmers.

2   Add the carrots and cook, stirring occasionally, until tender, about 5 minutes.

3   Add the chicken broth, coconut milk, lime zest, cumin, and salt. Stir in the potatoes and cod.

4   Bring to a boil and then reduce the heat to medium-low. Simmer until the potatoes are tender and the cod is cooked, about 20 minutes.

5   In a small bowl, whisk together the cornstarch and water. Add the mixture to the pot and cook, stirring constantly, until the stew thickens slightly, about 1 minute.

6   Stir in the cilantro and serve.

SUBSTITUTION TIP: *After the initial two weeks, if you aren't sensitive, feel free to add ½ cup of chopped red bell pepper along with the carrots.*

PER SERVING Calories: 277; Total Fat: 8g; Saturated Fat: 4g; Sodium: 619mg; Carbohydrates: 21g; Fiber: 2g; Protein: 30g

Linguine *with* Shrimp and Lemon

PREP TIME: 10 MINUTES / COOK TIME: 30 MINUTES

Many people love shrimp scampi, but with its high fat content and loads of garlic, it isn't the best choice for those with acid reflux. This version lowers the fat significantly and eliminates reflux-causing garlic while still offering delicious flavor. Serves 4

1 pound medium shrimp, shelled and deveined

1 cup Chicken Broth (page 185)

1 tablespoon extra-virgin olive oil

Zest of 1 lemon, grated

1 teaspoon Italian seasoning

½ teaspoon salt

½ cup bread crumbs

8 ounces linguine, cooked according to package directions

¼ cup chopped fresh parsley

1   Preheat the oven to 375°F.

2   Spread the shrimp in a single layer in a 9-by-13-inch baking pan.

3   In a small bowl, whisk together the chicken broth, olive oil, lemon zest, Italian seasoning, and salt. Pour the mixture over the shrimp.

4   Sprinkle the shrimp with the bread crumbs.

5   Bake until the shrimp turn pink and the bread crumbs are toasted, about 30 minutes.

6   Spoon the shrimp and liquid over the linguine, toss with the fresh parsley, and serve.

INGREDIENT TIP: *After the initial two weeks, if you aren't sensitive, try mixing ¼ cup grated Parmesan cheese into the bread crumbs.*

PER SERVING Calories: 369; Total Fat: 8g; Saturated Fat: 1g; Sodium: 854mg; Carbohydrates: 41g; Fiber: 1g; Protein: 34g

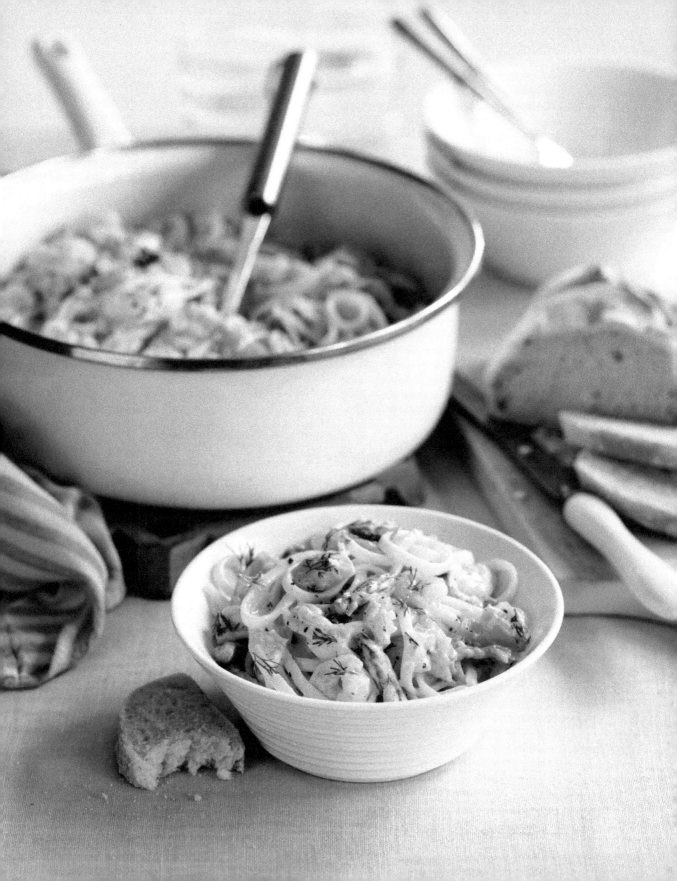

Linguine *with* Smoked Salmon and Shrimp

PREP TIME: 10 MINUTES / COOK TIME: 10 MINUTES

This linguine has a light cream sauce. Adding fresh dill complements the smoky-sweet flavor of the salmon and the shrimp, while lemon zest adds brightness. This is a dish that is best eaten fresh rather than reheated the next day. Serves 4

2 tablespoons extra-virgin olive oil

8 asparagus spears, chopped

6 ounces large shrimp, shelled and deveined

2 ounces smoked salmon, flaked

2 tablespoons all-purpose flour

2 cups nonfat milk

1 teaspoon grated lemon zest

½ teaspoon salt

8 ounces linguine, cooked according to package directions

2 tablespoons chopped fresh dill

1   In a large pot, heat the olive oil over medium-high heat until it shimmers.

2   Add the asparagus, shrimp, and smoked salmon. Cook, stirring occasionally, until the shrimp turn pink, about 4 minutes.

3   Remove the shrimp and salmon with a slotted spoon and transfer to a plate.

4   Add the flour to the pot and cook, stirring constantly, for 1 minute.

5   Stir in the milk, lemon zest, and salt. Cook, stirring constantly, until the sauce thickens, about 2 minutes.

6   In a large bowl, toss together the linguine, cooked shrimp and smoked salmon, sauce, and dill. Serve hot.

INGREDIENT TIP: *After the initial two weeks, if you aren't sensitive, add ¼ cup grated Parmesan cheese to each serving of pasta to add a savory cheesy flavor to the dish.*

PER SERVING Calories: 360; Total Fat: 10g; Saturated Fat: 2g; Sodium: 761mg; Carbohydrates: 43g; Fiber: 6g; Protein: 23g

Ginger-Glazed Scallops *with* Sugar Snap Peas

PREP TIME: 10 MINUTES / COOK TIME: 15 MINUTES

Scallops are sweet and earthy, but with a delicate texture. When paired with crisp sugar snap peas and a sweet-salty ginger glaze, they make a delicious main course. Because scallops are best when eaten just after cooking, this is definitely not a make-ahead dish. Serves 4

2 tablespoons extra-virgin olive oil, divided

1 pound sea scallops

1 teaspoon salt, divided

2 cups sugar snap peas

2 tablespoons grated fresh ginger

1 cup Chicken Broth (page 185)

1 tablespoon soy sauce

2 tablespoons honey

Zest of ½ orange, grated

1 tablespoon cornstarch

1 cup cooked brown rice

1   In a large skillet, heat 1 tablespoon of olive oil over medium-high heat until it shimmers.

2   Season the scallops with ½ teaspoon of salt and add them to the hot oil. Cook until done, about 2 minutes per side. Remove the scallops with tongs and transfer them to a platter.

3   In the same pan, heat the remaining 1 tablespoon of olive oil. Add the pea pods and ginger and cook, stirring occasionally, until the pea pods are soft, about 5 minutes.

4   In a small bowl, whisk together the chicken broth, soy sauce, honey, orange zest, cornstarch, and remaining ½ teaspoon of salt.

5   Add the mixture to the pan and cook, stirring constantly, until it begins to thicken, about 1 minute.

6   Return the scallops to the pan and turn them several times to coat them with the glaze.

7   Spoon over the brown rice and serve.

INGREDIENT TIP: *Scallops have a tendon that runs along the side that can be quite tough. Use a sharp knife to remove the tendon before cooking the scallops.*

PER SERVING Calories: 406; Total Fat: 10g; Saturated Fat: 2g; Sodium: 1,185mg; Carbohydrates: 54g; Fiber: 3g; Protein: 25g

Baked Cod *with* Ginger-Melon Salsa

PREP TIME: 10 MINUTES / COOK TIME: 15 MINUTES

Perfect for dinner on a hot summer evening, sweet cod is topped with a refreshing salsa made from honeydew melon. Citrus zest in both the salsa and the cod adds the flavor of acidity without heartburn-causing acid. Serves 4

4 (4-ounce) cod fillets

1 teaspoon salt, divided

Zest of 1 lemon, grated

2 tablespoons extra-virgin olive oil

Zest of 1 lime, grated

½ teaspoon ground cumin

2 cups small honeydew melon cubes

½ avocado, cubed

¼ cup chopped fresh cilantro

2 tablespoons grated fresh ginger

1 Preheat the oven to 400°F.

2 Line a baking sheet with parchment paper or aluminum foil.

3 Place the cod fillets on the lined baking sheet. Sprinkle them with ½ teaspoon of salt and the lemon zest.

4 Bake until the cod is opaque, about 15 minutes.

5 While the cod is baking, in a small bowl, whisk together the olive oil, lime zest, cumin, and remaining ½ teaspoon of salt.

6 Add the melon, avocado, cilantro, and ginger and toss well to combine.

7 Spoon the salsa over the cod and serve.

SUBSTITUTION TIP: *Although the recipe calls for cod, you can substitute any white fish, such as halibut or tilapia.*

PER SERVING Calories: 272; Total Fat: 13g; Saturated Fat: 2g; Sodium: 688mg; Carbohydrates: 12g; Fiber: 3g; Protein: 27g

Baked Halibut *with* Sour Cream-Dill Topping

PREP TIME: 10 MINUTES / COOK TIME: 25 MINUTES

Halibut is one of the mildest types of white fish. It is lightly sweet with firm yet flaky flesh. When you purchase halibut that is very fresh, it has almost no fishy odor or flavor, making it a favorite of people who are not usually fond of fish. Serves 4

1 pound halibut

½ teaspoon salt

1 cup nonfat sour cream

2 tablespoons chopped fresh dill

Zest of 1 lemon, grated

1   Preheat the oven to 350°F.

2   Line a baking sheet with parchment paper or aluminum foil.

3   Place the halibut on the lined sheet and sprinkle it with the salt.

4   In a small bowl, whisk together the sour cream, dill, and lemon zest.

5   Spread the mixture over the halibut.

6   Bake until the halibut is opaque and flakes easily, about 25 minutes. Serve.

INGREDIENT TIP: *If you aren't sensitive to red bell peppers, cook ¼ cup finely chopped red bell peppers in 1 tablespoon of olive oil until soft and add them to the sour cream mixture.*

PER SERVING Calories: 183; Total Fat: 1g; Saturated Fat: 0g; Sodium: 432mg; Carbohydrates: 11g; Fiber: 0g; Protein: 28g

Creamy Rice *with* Shrimp, Peas, and Basil

PREP TIME: 10 MINUTES / COOK TIME: 15 MINUTES

While authentic risotto is pretty labor intensive with all that stirring, this recipe mimics the creamy texture of the dish without most of the effort. Use precooked rice to save time. Serves 4

2 tablespoons extra-virgin olive oil

2 ounces turkey bacon, cut into pieces

12 ounces medium shrimp, peeled and deveined

1 cup peas (fresh or frozen)

1 tablespoon all-purpose flour

1 cup nonfat milk

1 teaspoon grated lemon zest

1 teaspoon salt

1½ cups cooked brown rice

¼ small fresh basil leaves or chopped fresh basil

1   In a large pot or skillet, heat the olive oil over medium-high heat until it shimmers.

2   Add the turkey bacon and cook, stirring occasionally, until browned, about 4 minutes.

3   Add the shrimp and peas and cook, stirring occasionally, until the shrimp are pink, about 4 minutes.

4   Add the flour and cook, stirring constantly, for 30 seconds.

5   Stir in the milk, lemon zest, and salt and cook until the mixture thickens, about 1 minute.

6   Stir in the rice and cook until it is heated through, a minute or two more. Stir in the basil and serve.

INGREDIENT TIP: *If you like your risotto cheesy, add ¼ cup of grated Parmesan cheese after the sauce thickens and cook, stirring constantly, until the cheese is completely melted, about 1 minute.*

PER SERVING Calories: 492; Total Fat: 10g; Saturated Fat: 2g; Sodium: 936mg; Carbohydrates: 67g; Fiber: 3g; Protein: 31g

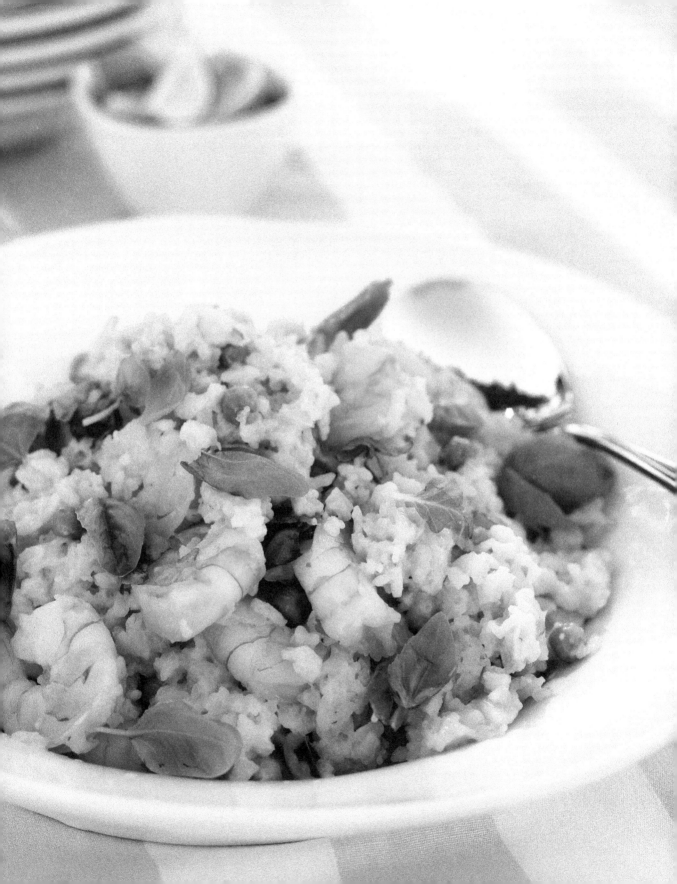

Maple-Soy Glazed Salmon

**PREP TIME: 5 MINUTES, PLUS 10 MINUTES FOR MARINATING /
COOK TIME: 25 MINUTES**

Salmon is loaded with healthy omega-3 fatty acids. Wild-caught Pacific salmon is the most flavorful and healthy type of salmon. Cook with the skin on, but remove before serving. This dish goes well with brown rice and Honey-Roasted Asparagus (page 100). Serves 4

¼ cup Chicken Broth (page 185)

¼ cup soy sauce

¼ cup pure maple syrup

4 (4-ounce) salmon fillets

1 Preheat the oven to 425°F.

2 Line a baking sheet with parchment paper or aluminum foil.

3 In a shallow dish, whisk together the chicken broth, soy sauce, and maple syrup.

4 Put the salmon, flesh-side down, in the mixture and allow it to marinate for 10 minutes.

5 Remove the salmon from the marinade and place it, flesh-side up, on the lined baking sheet. Transfer the marinade to a small saucepan.

6 Bake the salmon until it is opaque and flakes easily, about 25 minutes.

7 While the salmon bakes, bring the marinade to a boil over medium-high heat. Reduce the heat to medium-low and simmer, stirring frequently, until it is syrupy, about 5 minutes.

8 Brush the syrup over the baked salmon and turn on the broiler. Put the salmon under the broiler for about 2 minutes to harden the glaze slightly. Serve.

INGREDIENT TIP: *When buying salmon or other fish, look for fish with firm, clear flesh. The fish should smell like seawater and not overtly fishy.*

PER SERVING Calories: 212; Total Fat: 7g; Saturated Fat: 1g; Sodium: 998mg; Carbohydrates: 15g; Fiber: 0g; Protein: 23g

Honey-Ginger Salmon

PREP TIME: 10 MINUTES / COOK TIME: 30 MINUTES

The lightly spicy flavor of ginger works nicely with the sweet flesh of the salmon, especially when there's honey in the glaze as well. Serve this with baked butternut squash and a small side of brown rice for a satisfying meal that won't aggravate your acid reflux. Serves 4

¼ cup Chicken Broth (page 185)

¼ cup honey

2 tablespoons grated fresh ginger

Zest of 1 orange, grated

½ teaspoon salt

4 (4-ounce) salmon fillets

1   Preheat the oven to 425°F.

2   Line a baking sheet with parchment paper or aluminum foil.

3   In a shallow dish, whisk together the chicken broth, honey, ginger, orange zest, and salt.

4   Put the salmon, flesh-side down, in the mixture and allow it to marinate for 10 minutes.

5   Remove the salmon from the marinade and place it, flesh-side up, on the lined baking sheet. Transfer the marinade to a small saucepan.

6   Bake the salmon until it is opaque and flakes easily, about 25 minutes.

7   While the salmon bakes, bring the marinade to a boil over medium-high heat. Reduce the heat to medium-low and simmer, stirring frequently, until it is syrupy, about 5 minutes.

8   Brush the syrup over the baked salmon and turn on the broiler. Put the salmon under the broiler for about 2 minutes to harden the glaze slightly. Serve.

INGREDIENT TIP: *To grate fresh ginger, use a sharp knife or peeler to remove the fibrous brown outer skin. Then, use a rasp-style grater to yield finely grated bits of ginger.*

PER SERVING Calories: 226; Total Fat: 7g; Saturated Fat: 1g; Sodium: 390mg; Carbohydrates: 20g; Fiber: 0g; Protein: 23g

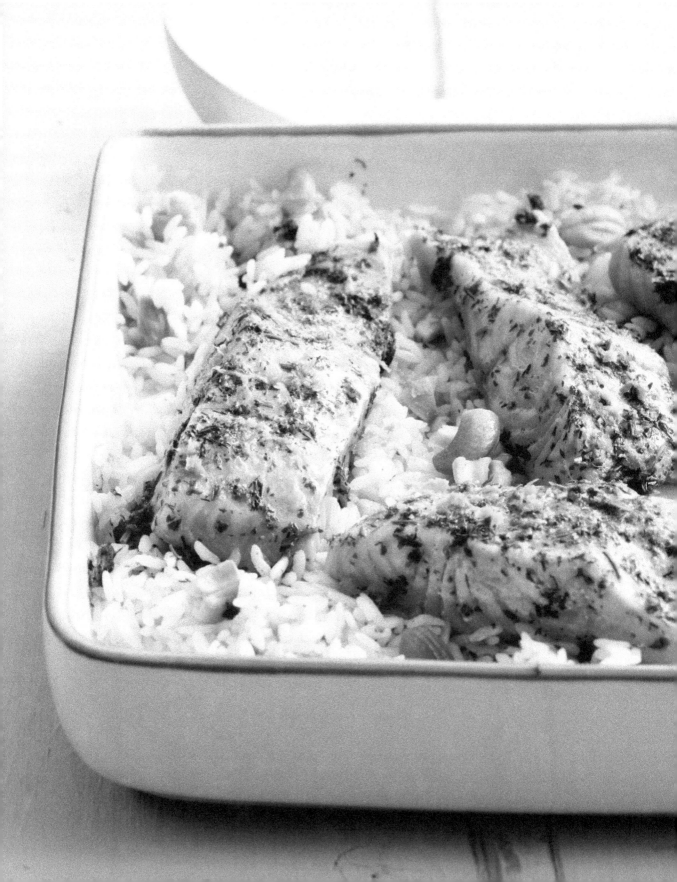

Orange Salmon *with* Cashew Rice

PREP TIME: 10 MINUTES / COOK TIME: 40 MINUTES

This simple one-dish meal cooks quickly in the oven. To save time, use precooked rice. Cashews are high in fat, but this recipe uses only a very small amount, so it shouldn't aggravate your GERD. If you are sensitive to cashews, you can leave them out completely. Serves 4

1 cup cooked brown rice

¼ cup cashews, chopped

4 (4-ounce) salmon fillets

¼ cup Chicken Broth (page 185)

2 tablespoons honey

Zest of 2 oranges, grated

¼ cup chopped fresh parsley

2 tablespoons chopped fresh dill

½ teaspoon salt

1. Preheat the oven to 350°F.

2. In a shallow baking dish, mix together the rice and cashews.

3. Lay the salmon fillets, flesh-side up, on top of the rice.

4. In a small bowl, whisk together the chicken broth, honey, orange zest, parsley, dill, and salt. Pour the mixture over the top of the salmon fillets.

5. Bake until the salmon is opaque and flakes easily, 30 to 40 minutes.

6. Place a portion of the cashew rice and a salmon fillet on each plate and serve.

SUBSTITUTION TIP: *For a more delicate flavor, replace the salmon with halibut fillets.*

PER SERVING Calories: 408; Total Fat: 12g; Saturated Fat: 2g; Sodium: 398mg; Carbohydrates: 50g; Fiber: 1g; Protein: 27g

Tuna Noodle Casserole

PREP TIME: 15 MINUTES / COOK TIME: 1 HOUR AND 10 MINUTES

Tuna noodle casserole is tasty, but it's also usually loaded with fat. This recipe minimizes the fat but still offers the delicious tuna casserole flavor you remember from when you were a kid. *Serves 4*

Nonstick cooking spray

1 (6-ounce) can water-packed tuna, drained

1 cup peas (fresh or frozen)

1 cup cooked whole-wheat macaroni

2 tablespoons extra-virgin olive oil

8 ounces cremini mushrooms, quartered

1 teaspoon chopped fresh thyme

2 tablespoons all-purpose flour

1 cup Chicken Broth (page 185)

1 cup nonfat milk

Zest of 1 lemon, grated

1 teaspoon salt

½ cup bread crumbs

1   Preheat the oven to 350°F.

2   Spray a 9-inch square baking pan with nonstick cooking spray.

3   In a medium bowl, combine the tuna, peas, and macaroni. Set aside.

4   In a large skillet, heat the olive oil over medium-high heat until it shimmers.

5   Add the mushrooms and thyme and cook, stirring occasionally, until the mushrooms are golden brown, about 6 minutes.

6   Add the flour and cook, stirring constantly, for 1 minute. Stir in the chicken broth, milk, lemon zest, and salt. Stir continuously until the mixture simmers and thickens, about 4 minutes. Pour over the tuna mixture. Stir to combine.

7   Spread the mixture evenly in the prepared pan. Sprinkle with the bread crumbs. Bake until hot and bubbly, about 1 hour. Serve warm.

SUBSTITUTION TIP: *If you aren't sensitive to cheese, you can add ¼ cup grated sharp cheddar cheese to the mixture just before spreading it in the pan.*

PER SERVING Calories: 346; Total Fat: 9g; Saturated Fat: 2g; Sodium: 961mg; Carbohydrates: 43g; Fiber: 5g; Protein: 24g

Southwestern Shrimp, Mushrooms, and Rice

PREP TIME: 10 MINUTES / COOK TIME: 30 MINUTES

It's easy to make this dish because you quickly throw the ingredients into a baking pan and sit down to a delicious meal just 30 minutes later. While the recipe calls for cooked brown rice, you can also serve the stew atop fresh pasta. Serves 4

1 pound medium shrimp, shelled and deveined

8 ounces button mushrooms, halved

1 cup peas (fresh or frozen)

2 tablespoons extra-virgin olive oil

Zest of 1 lime, grated

1 teaspoon ground cumin

½ teaspoon salt

¼ cup chopped fresh cilantro

1 cup cooked brown rice

1   Preheat the oven to 375°F.

2   In a bowl, toss together the shrimp, mushrooms, peas, olive oil, lime zest, cumin, and salt until combined.

3   Spread the shrimp mixture in a single layer in a 9-by-13-inch baking pan.

4   Bake until the shrimp turn pink and the mushrooms are soft, about 30 minutes.

5   Stir in the cilantro. Spoon over the rice to serve.

INGREDIENT TIP: *To devein shrimp, run a sharp knife along the curved spine of the shrimp and pull out the small vein that runs along it.*

PER SERVING Calories: 384; Total Fat: 10g; Saturated Fat: 1g; Sodium: 555mg; Carbohydrates: 44g; Fiber: 4g; Protein: 32g

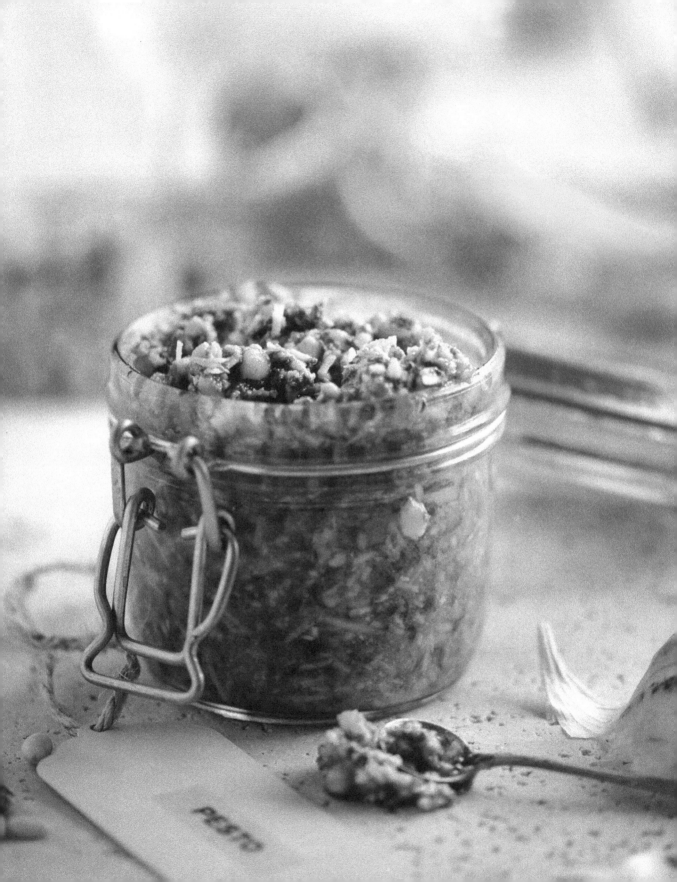

Chapter Ten

Broths, Sauces, and Condiments

Vegetable Broth

PREP TIME: 10 MINUTES / COOK TIME: 30 MINUTES

Making your own vegetable broth ensures you won't get any heartburn-inducing veggies in it. This broth is unsalted so that you can control the level of salt in your recipes. You can store the broth for up to 6 months in the freezer, tightly sealed in 1-cup serving portions. Makes 6 cups

1 cup chopped carrots
(or carrot peels)

1 cup chopped celery (or celery trimmings, including leaves)

1 cup chopped fennel (or fennel trimmings, including fronds)

1 cup chopped mushrooms

8 cups water

1 fresh rosemary sprig

2 fresh thyme sprigs

2 bay leaves

1   In a large stockpot, combine all of the ingredients.

2   Bring the mixture to a boil over medium-high heat and then reduce the heat to medium-low. Simmer for 30 minutes. Feel free to add more water if evaporation causes the broth to reduce to less than 6 cups.

3   Set a fine-mesh sieve over a bowl and carefully pour the stock through it, straining out the solids.

COOKING TIP: *There's no need to waste your vegetable trimmings by throwing them away. Instead, save them in a resealable bag in the freezer to use when you're making broth. Vegetable trimmings good for broth include carrot peels and ends, fennel trimmings, zucchini peels, celery trimmings, asparagus ends, and mushroom stems. Avoid using cruciferous veggie trimmings like broccoli or cauliflower, which will impart too strong of a flavor to the broth.*

PER SERVING (1 CUP) Calories: 38; Total Fat: 1g; Saturated Fat: 0g; Sodium: 763mg; Carbohydrates: 1g; Fiber: 0g; Protein: 5g

Chicken Broth

PREP TIME: 10 MINUTES / COOK TIME: 3 HOURS

Even though this broth is rendered from skin-on chicken, it remains low-fat because for the final step, you skim all the fat from the broth. As noted in the vegetable broth recipe, you can use an array of vegetable trimmings in your broth to give it flavor. Makes 6 cups

3 pounds chicken wings

2 carrots, roughly chopped

2 celery stalks, roughly chopped

2 cups chopped mushrooms

8 cups water

2 fresh rosemary sprigs

2 fresh thyme sprigs

1 bay leaf

1   In a large stockpot, combine all of the ingredients.

2   Bring the mixture to a boil over medium-high heat and then reduce the heat to medium-low. Simmer for 3 hours, stirring very occasionally. Feel free to add more water if evaporation causes the broth to reduce to less than 6 cups.

3   Set a fine-mesh sieve over a bowl and carefully pour the stock through it, straining out the solids.

4   Cover and refrigerate the broth overnight.

5   In the morning, skim all the solidified fat off the top of the broth, discarding the fat and reserving the broth.

COOKING TIP: *If you don't want to waste perfectly good chicken parts on broth, it's okay. You can also save the bones from cooked chicken in a resealable bag in your freezer. All bones, including the carcass of a roasted chicken, contribute to a flavorful stock.*

PER SERVING (1 CUP) Calories: 38; Total Fat: 1g; Saturated Fat: 0g; Sodium: 763mg; Carbohydrates: 1g; Fiber: 0g; Protein: 5g

Ginger-Lime Vinaigrette

PREP TIME: 5 MINUTES / COOK TIME: 0

This vinaigrette is delicious for topping steamed veggies or a salad. It also serves as a delicious marinade for chicken breasts. Remember the 1-tablespoon per day restriction. Because it contains vinegar, if you eat too much it can trigger acid reflux. Serves 6

¼ cup extra-virgin olive oil

2 tablespoons apple cider vinegar

Zest of 1 lime, grated

1 tablespoon grated fresh ginger

1 teaspoon Dijon mustard

¼ teaspoon salt

In a small bowl, whisk together all of the ingredients until combined. Whisk again before using.

INGREDIENT TIP: *In vinaigrettes, mustard works as an emulsifier to help keep the oil and vinegar mixed together.*

PER SERVING (1 TABLESPOON) Calories: 77; Total Fat: 8g; Saturated Fat: 1g; Sodium: 107mg; Carbohydrates: 1g; Fiber: 0g; Protein: 0g

Orange-Honey-Dijon Dressing

PREP TIME: 5 MINUTES / COOK TIME: 0

Spread this dressing on pork tenderloin or chicken breasts, or use it on a salad. It's also a delicious dipping sauce for Baked Chicken Tenders (page 147), or ideal as a spread for sandwiches or turkey burgers.

Serves 8

¼ cup plain nonfat Greek yogurt

2 tablespoons honey

2 tablespoons Dijon mustard

1 teaspoon grated orange zest

¼ teaspoon salt

In a small bowl, whisk together all of the ingredients until combined.

SUBSTITUTION TIP: *For a dairy-free version, replace the yogurt with silken tofu that has been blended in the blender with 2 tablespoons of water until smooth.*

PER SERVING (1 TABLESPOON) Calories: 23; Total Fat: 0g; Saturated Fat: 0g; Sodium: 124mg; Carbohydrates: 5g; Fiber: 0g; Protein: 0g

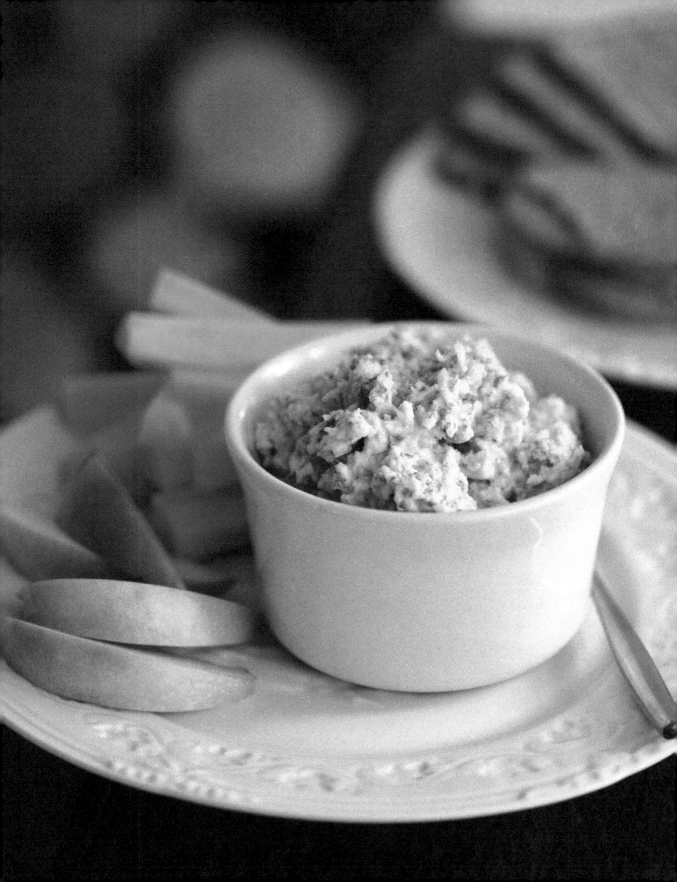

Creamy Herb Dip

PREP TIME: 5 MINUTES / COOK TIME: 0

This makes a tasty sandwich spread, or it is equally delicious as a dip for sliced vegetables. Feel free to change the herbs to suit your own tastes in this delicious dip. Serves 8

½ cup plain nonfat Greek yogurt

1 cup baby arugula

2 tablespoons chopped fresh thyme

¼ cup chopped fresh basil

1 teaspoon grated lemon zest

½ teaspoon salt

In a blender, combine all of the ingredients. Blend on high until smooth, about 30 seconds.

SUBSTITUTION TIP: *For a slightly tangier dip, replace the Greek yogurt with nonfat sour cream.*

PER SERVING (2 TABLESPOONS) Calories: 11; Total Fat: 0g; Saturated Fat: 0g; Sodium: 160mg; Carbohydrates: 2g; Fiber: 1g; Protein: 1g

Creamy Ranch Dressing

PREP TIME: 5 MINUTES / COOK TIME: 0

Looking for a tasty ranch dressing to use as a salad topper, sandwich spread, or dip? This dressing will fit the bill. It's also tasty as a low-fat topping for baked russet or sweet potatoes. This dressing will store in the refrigerator, tightly sealed, for up to 3 days. Serves 5

¼ cup plain nonfat Greek yogurt

1 tablespoon Dijon mustard

2 teaspoons grated lemon zest

1 teaspoons dried dill

½ teaspoon dried thyme

¼ teaspoon salt

In a small bowl, whisk together all of the ingredients until combined.

SUBSTITUTION TIP: *If you wish, stir in 2 tablespoons of grated Parmesan cheese.*

PER SERVING (1 tablespoon) Calories: 10; Total Fat: 0g; Saturated Fat: 0g; Sodium: 161mg; Carbohydrates: 2g; Fiber: 0g; Protein: 1g

Lemon and Artichoke Pesto

PREP TIME: 5 MINUTES / COOK TIME: 0

This sauce is so easy, and yet so delicious. It's tasty as a pasta topping, or you can spread it on fish, poultry, or meat. It even makes a tasty spread for bread or dip for vegetables. If you love artichokes, you'll love this pesto. Makes 1 cup

1 (14-ounce) can artichoke hearts, drained

2 tablespoons grated lemon zest

½ cup loosely packed fresh basil leaves

2 tablespoons extra-virgin olive oil

1 tablespoon pine nuts

¼ cup grated Parmesan cheese

¼ teaspoon salt

In a blender or food processor, pulse all of the ingredients until well chopped and combined, about ten 1-second pulses.

SUBSTITUTION TIP: *To reduce the fat content, eliminate the Parmesan cheese and pine nuts and reduce the olive oil to 1 tablespoon.*

PER SERVING (2 TABLESPOONS) Calories: 88; Total Fat: 6g; Saturated Fat: 2g; Sodium: 169mg; Carbohydrates: 7g; Fiber: 4g; Protein: 4g

Butternut Squash Chutney

PREP TIME: 20 MINUTES / COOK TIME: 40 MINUTES

Chutney is a wonderful spread for bread or toast. You can also use it as a fruit or vegetable dip, or to top fish, poultry, or meat. This versatile blend is fragrant with ginger and orange zest, and has a delicious flavor. Makes 1 cup

½ butternut squash, peeled and finely chopped

1 apple, cored, peeled, and finely chopped

Zest of 1 orange, grated

1 teaspoon grated fresh ginger

½ cup water

2 tablespoons apple cider vinegar

½ teaspoon salt

¼ teaspoon ground cloves

¼ teaspoon chopped fresh rosemary (optional)

¼ cup sugar

1 In a large pot, combine all of the ingredients and bring to a boil over medium-high heat.

2 Reduce the heat to medium-low and continue cooking, stirring occasionally, until the fruit and vegetables are soft and the liquid is a syrup, about 40 minutes.

3 Cool before serving.

SUBSTITUTION TIP: *You can also use pumpkin flesh in this recipe, which will give it a slightly earthier flavor.*

PER SERVING (2 TABLESPOONS) Calories: 21; Total Fat: 0g; Saturated Fat: 0g; Sodium: 74mg; Carbohydrates: 5g; Fiber: 0g; Protein: 0g

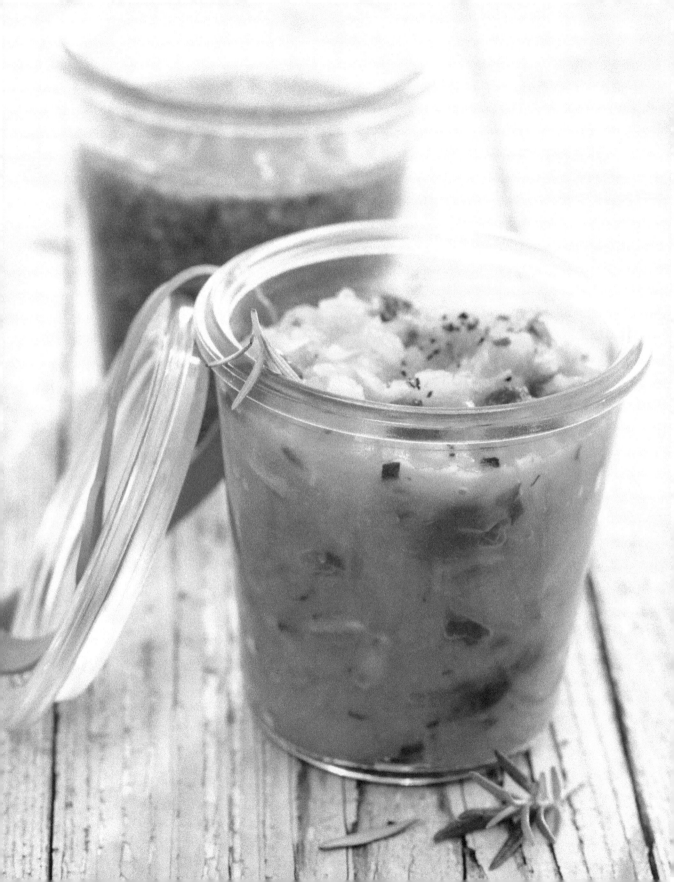

Coconut-Pumpkin Dip

PREP TIME: 5 MINUTES / COOK TIME: 0

This sweet dip is delicious as a bread spread, or as a dip for apples or pears. The coconut milk makes the dip creamy, while the pumpkin has a sweet yet earthy flavor. Adding fragrant spices elevates the flavor profile of the dip. Makes 1 cup

¾ cup canned pumpkin purée

¼ cup light coconut milk

2 tablespoons brown sugar

½ teaspoon grated orange zest

½ teaspoon ground ginger

½ teaspoon ground cinnamon

Pinch ground cloves

Pinch salt

In a small bowl, whisk together all of the ingredients until well blended. Chill before serving.

INGREDIENT TIP: *Make sure you purchase pure pumpkin purée, and not pumpkin pie filling. The pie mix already has cream and spices mixed into it.*

PER SERVING (2 TABLESPOONS) Calories: 17; Total Fat: 1g; Saturated Fat: 1g; Sodium: 13mg; Carbohydrates: 2g; Fiber: 0g; Protein: 0g

Mediterranean Chickpea Spread

PREP TIME: 5 MINUTES / COOK TIME: 0

Use this as a sandwich spread or a dip for fresh veggies. It has delicious Mediterranean herbs and spices, so it adds a savory flavor to anything in which you use it. Makes 1 cup

½ cup plain nonfat Greek yogurt

½ cup canned chickpeas, rinsed and drained

½ teaspoon toasted sesame oil

½ teaspoon ground cumin

1 teaspoon grated lemon zest

½ teaspoon salt

In a blender, combine all of the ingredients. Blend on high until smooth, about 30 seconds.

SUBSTITUTION TIP: *You can substitute canned white beans or black beans for the chickpeas in this recipe.*

PER SERVING (2 TABLESPOONS) Calories: 57; Total Fat: 1g; Saturated Fat: 0g; Sodium: 162mg; Carbohydrates: 9g; Fiber: 2g; Protein: 3g

Low-Fat Mayonnaise Replacement

PREP TIME: 5 MINUTES / COOK TIME: 0

Mayonnaise is a popular spread, but it is very high in fat. Nonfat Greek yogurt is creamy and light, making it the perfect base for a mayonnaise spread, while puréed tofu gives it more spreadability. The combination makes a tasty mayo substitute for sandwiches.
Serves 8

½ cup plain nonfat Greek yogurt

½ cup silken tofu

½ teaspoon fish sauce

½ teaspoon grated lemon zest

1 teaspoon apple cider vinegar

¼ teaspoon salt

In a blender, combine all of the ingredients. Blend on high until smooth, about 1 minute.

SUBSTITUTION TIP: *To go completely vegan with this, replace the fish sauce with soy sauce and the yogurt with soy yogurt.*

PER SERVING (2 TABLESPOONS) Calories: 20; Total Fat: 1g; Saturated Fat: 0g; Sodium: 116mg; Carbohydrates: 2g; Fiber: 0g; Protein: 2g

Southwestern Avocado Spread

PREP TIME: 5 MINUTES / COOK TIME: 0

You can use this as a dip for vegetables, or to make a sandwich or burger more interesting. Although avocados are a bit high in fat, they are really soothing for acid reflux. With added southwestern spices, this is a tasty spread or dip. Serves 4

½ avocado

2 tablespoons plain nonfat Greek yogurt

2 tablespoons chopped fresh cilantro

Zest of 1 lime, grated

½ teaspoon ground cumin

½ teaspoon ground coriander

¼ teaspoon salt

1   In a small bowl, mash the avocado with a fork until smooth.

2   Stir in the yogurt, cilantro, lime zest, cumin, coriander, and salt.

INGREDIENT TIP: *To store this without the avocados going brown, put plastic wrap directly on the surface of the spread so no air can reach it. Then, seal the container.*

PER SERVING (2 TABLESPOONS) Calories: 57; Total Fat: 5g; Saturated Fat: 1g; Sodium: 155mg; Carbohydrates: 3g; Fiber: 2g; Protein: 1g

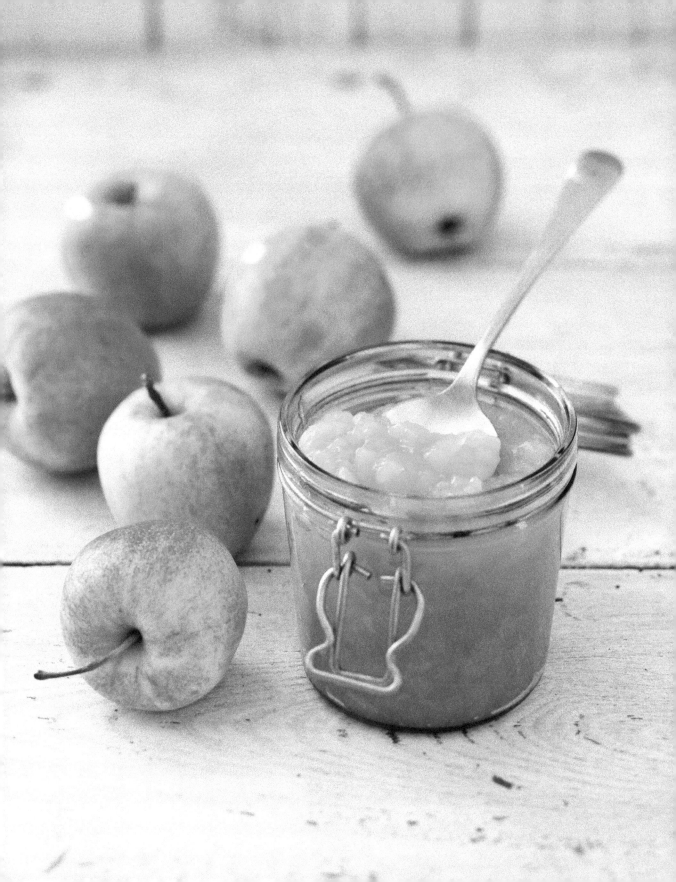

Applesauce with Fennel and Ginger

PREP TIME: 10 MINUTES / COOK TIME: 20 MINUTES

This applesauce isn't your traditional applesauce. Instead, it has two tummy-calming ingredients—fennel and ginger—so it's a wonderful sauce for poultry, pork tenderloin, or fish. You can serve it as a tasty side dish. Serves 4

2 tablespoons extra-virgin olive oil

½ fennel bulb, trimmed and thinly sliced

1 tablespoon grated fresh ginger

2 red apples, such as Fuji, peeled, cored, and sliced

¼ cup water

2 tablespoons pure maple syrup

Pinch salt

1   In a large skillet, heat the olive oil over medium-high heat until it shimmers.

2   Add the fennel and ginger and cook, stirring occasionally, until it softens, about 5 minutes.

3   Add the apples and cook, stirring occasionally, until they begin to soften, about 5 minutes more.

4   Add the water, maple syrup, and salt. Cook, occasionally using the back of the spoon to press on the apples and turn them into sauce, until the apples are very soft, about 10 minutes more. Serve warm or chilled.

COOKING TIP: *This sauce has a rustic, slightly chunky texture. If you'd like a smoother sauce, then purée it in a blender before serving.*

PER SERVING Calories: 165; Total Fat: 7g; Saturated Fat: 1g; Sodium: 56mg; Carbohydrates: 27g; Fiber: 4g; Protein: 1g

Tropical Black Bean Salsa

PREP TIME: 10 MINUTES / COOK TIME: 0

This tasty salsa tastes great on grilled fish or chicken, or it's delicious to serve as a dip for veggies or crackers. Try dipping sliced jicama in this salsa for a tasty snack. This doesn't keep well because of the bananas, so it is best if it's made fresh. Serves 4

1 banana, peeled and chopped

½ cup chopped cantaloupe

½ cup canned black beans, rinsed and drained

¼ cup chopped fresh cilantro

Zest of 1 lime, grated

½ teaspoon ground cumin

½ teaspoon salt

In a small bowl, combine all of the ingredients.

INGREDIENT TIP: *If you like, you can replace the banana with cubed avocado, which also works well in this salsa.*

PER SERVING (½ CUP) Calories: 117; Total Fat: 1g; Saturated Fat: 0g; Sodium: 296mg; Carbohydrates: 24g; Fiber: 5g; Protein: 6g

Low-Fat Alfredo Sauce

PREP TIME: 5 MINUTES / COOK TIME: 10 MINUTES

Alfredo sauce is a delicious pasta topping as well as a wonderful sauce for fish or poultry. It is, however, typically laden with fat in the form of whole milk, butter, and heavy cream. This version removes all of the fatty ingredients (with the exception of a little butter and Parmesan), making it much lighter and acid-reflux friendly. Serves 4

1 tablespoon unsalted butter

1 tablespoons all-purpose flour

1 cup nonfat milk

¼ teaspoon ground nutmeg

¼ teaspoon salt

¼ cup grated Parmesan cheese

1   In a large saucepan, melt the butter over medium-high heat.

2   Add the flour and cook, stirring constantly, for 1 minute.

3   Add the milk, nutmeg, and salt and cook, stirring constantly, until the sauce thickens, 3 to 4 minutes more.

4   Reduce the heat to low. Stir in the Parmesan cheese. Cook, stirring constantly, until the cheese melts, 2 to 3 minutes.

SUBSTITUTION TIP: *For a yellow cheese version, as you'd find on mac and cheese, replace the Parmesan cheese with grated sharp cheddar cheese.*

PER SERVING (¼ CUP) Calories: 101; Total Fat: 6g; Saturated Fat: 4g; Sodium: 332mg; Carbohydrates: 5g; Fiber: 0g; Protein: 7g

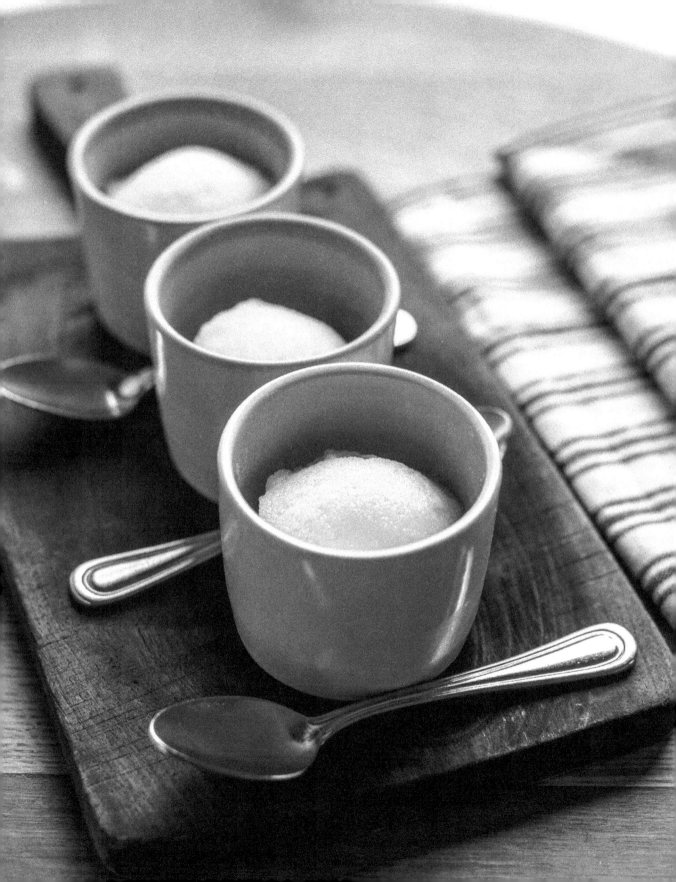

Chapter Eleven

Desserts and Sweets

Honeydew Sorbet

**PREP TIME: 20 MINUTES, PLUS ABOUT 5 HOURS FOR CHILLING /
COOK TIME: 5 MINUTES**

This sweet sorbet is lightly flavored and very refreshing. It makes a delicious dessert, or you can use it as a palate cleanser or tasty snack on a hot afternoon. This sorbet is tastiest when honeydew melons are in season in the mid to late spring. Serves 4

½ cup water

¼ cup honey

¼ cup sugar

1 honeydew melon, peeled and cubed

1   In a small saucepan, stir the water, honey, and sugar over medium-high heat until the sugar dissolves completely. Cool the mixture.

2   In a blender, combine the honeydew melon and the cooled syrup. Process until smooth.

3   Pour the mixture into a 9-inch square baking dish. Freeze for 1 hour.

4   Using a fork, scrape the mixture to distribute the ice crystals. Return the dish to the freezer.

5   Repeat steps 3 and 4 about five times, until the granita is completely frozen. Serve.

SUBSTITUTION TIP: *For a slightly sweeter flavor, try replacing the honeydew with an equal amount of cantaloupe.*

PER SERVING Calories: 227; Total Fat: 1g; Saturated Fat: 0g; Sodium: 4mg; Carbohydrates: 59g; Fiber: 3g; Protein: 2g

Creamy Cantaloupe Ice Pops

PREP TIME: 5 MINUTES, PLUS 12 HOURS FOR CHILLING / COOK TIME: 0

Ice pops make a fantastic and portable dessert. If you have ice pop molds, great! If not, however, you don't need to worry. You can also freeze the pops in paper cups with wooden sticks. Just put aluminum foil over the top of the cup and push the stick through it to hold it in place. Serves 6

1 cantaloupe, peeled and cubed

1 cup light coconut milk

½ cup plain nonfat yogurt

2 tablespoons honey

¼ teaspoon ground cinnamon

1   Combine all of the ingredients in a blender and blend until smooth.

2   Pour the mixture into six ice pop holders or paper cups.

3   Freeze for 12 hours, or until set. Serve.

COOKING TIP: *If you use paper cups, it is unlikely you'll be able to remove the ice pop from the cup. However, it is easy to peel away the cup from around the ice pop when you're ready to serve them.*

PER SERVING Calories: 64; Total Fat: 3g; Saturated Fat: 2g; Sodium: 31mg; Carbohydrates: 11g; Fiber: 0g; Protein: 2g

Coffee Granita

PREP TIME: 20 MINUTES, PLUS ABOUT 5 HOURS FOR CHILLING /
COOK TIME: 5 MINUTES

This frozen sweet coffee dessert doesn't require any special equipment—just a saucepan, a baking dish, and a fork. Since having more than about a cup of coffee a day is an invitation to acid reflux, have this in place of your daily cup of joe for a sweet dessert. Serves 4

1 cup strong brewed
decaffeinated coffee

¼ cup brown sugar

½ teaspoon grated orange zest

1 In a small saucepan, stir the coffee, brown sugar, and orange zest over medium-high heat until the sugar dissolves.

2 Pour the mixture into a 9-inch square baking dish.

3 Freeze for about 1 hour.

4 Using a fork, scrape the granita to distribute the ice crystals. Return the pan to the freezer.

5 Repeat steps 3 and 4 about five times, until the granita is completely frozen. Serve.

SUBSTITUTION TIP: *For a different flavoring, consider using 1 teaspoon of flavored syrup in place of or in addition to the orange zest.*

PER SERVING Calories: 35; Total Fat: 0g; Saturated Fat: 0g; Sodium: 4mg; Carbohydrates: 9g; Fiber: 0g; Protein: 0g

Maple-Banana Milkshake

PREP TIME: 5 MINUTES / COOK TIME: 0

This tasty milkshake offers more than bananas. It is also sweetly scented with fragrant cinnamon and warm maple. For best results, freeze the bananas before using. Serves 2

1 banana, peeled and cut into pieces and frozen

1 cup nonfat milk

½ cup nonfat vanilla frozen yogurt

2 tablespoons pure maple syrup

1 teaspoon ground cinnamon

Combine all of the ingredients in a blender and blend until smooth. Serve right away.

SUBSTITUTION TIP: *To make this dairy-free, use rice milk and low-fat rice or frozen soy yogurt.*

PER SERVING Calories: 208; Total Fat: 0g; Saturated Fat: 0g; Sodium: 100mg; Carbohydrates: 46g; Fiber: 2g; Protein: 6g

Gingered Baked Pears

PREP TIME: 5 MINUTES / COOK TIME: 30 MINUTES

Ginger, honey, and cinnamon take pears from ordinary to extraordinary. This recipe is best in the fall, when pears are at the peak of their ripeness. If you like, serve with a small scoop of nonfat vanilla frozen yogurt or ice cream. Serves 4

2 pears, halved

½ teaspoon ground cinnamon

½ teaspoon ground ginger

1 tablespoon honey

1 Preheat the oven to 350°F.

2 Use a spoon or melon baller to remove the core of each pear half.

3 Place the pears in a 9-inch square baking dish.

4 Sprinkle the pears with the cinnamon and ginger and drizzle them with the honey.

5 Bake until the pears are soft, about 30 minutes. Serve warm.

SUBSTITUTION TIP: *You can replace the honey with pure maple syrup to give the pears a warmer flavor profile.*

PER SERVING (½ PEAR) Calories: 78; Total Fat: 0g; Saturated Fat: 0g; Sodium: 2mg; Carbohydrates: 21g; Fiber: 3g; Protein: 0g

Chilled Melon Soup *with* Ginger

PREP TIME: 10 MINUTES / COOK TIME: 0

This sweetly refreshing soup combines cool cantaloupe with tummy-soothing ginger and honey. With a little added spice, the soup is the perfect dessert for an early summer evening when cantaloupes are at their peak of ripeness. Serves 4

½ cantaloupe, peeled and roughly chopped

½ cup plain nonfat yogurt

½ cup nonfat milk

2 tablespoons grated fresh ginger

1 tablespoon honey

1 teaspoon grated orange zest

¼ teaspoon ground nutmeg

Combine all of the ingredients in a blender and process until smooth. Serve chilled.

SUBSTITUTION TIP: *Honeydew melon also works well in this delicious soup, giving it a sweeter flavor.*

PER SERVING Calories: 57; Total Fat: 0g; Saturated Fat: 0g; Sodium: 39mg; Carbohydrates: 11g; Fiber: 1g; Protein: 3g

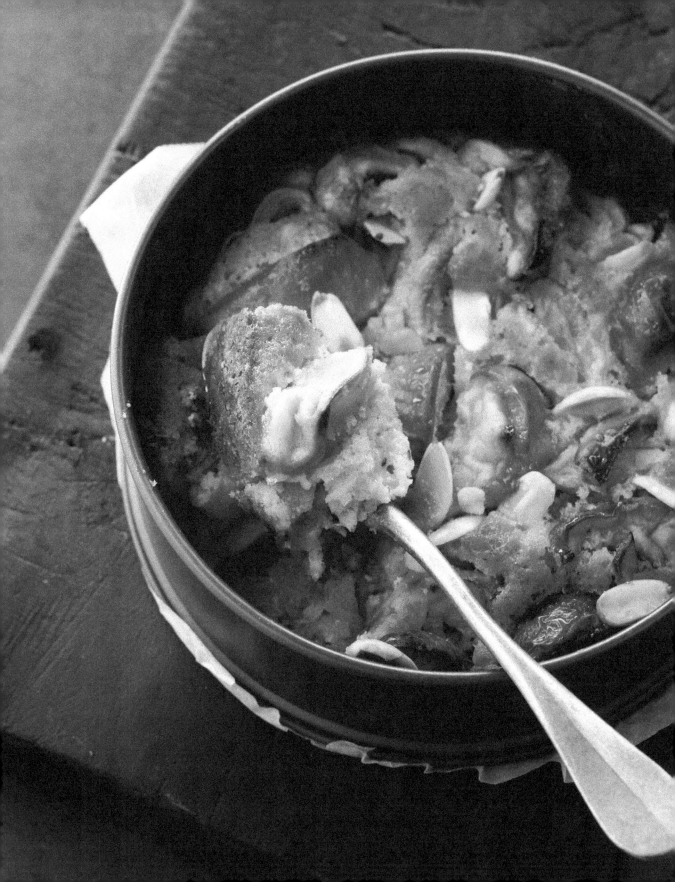

Baked Apple Pudding

PREP TIME: 15 MINUTES, PLUS 1 HOUR FOR CHILLING /
COOK TIME: 45 MINUTES

This bread pudding is creamy and delicious. With sweet apples and fragrant cinnamon in a tasty custard, it tastes sinful but it won't aggravate your GERD. It also keeps well, and even gets better after a few days, so it's a great make-ahead dessert. Serves 6

Nonstick cooking spray

2 cups nonfat milk

3 large eggs, beaten

¼ cup pure maple syrup

½ cup sugar

1 teaspoon grated fresh ginger

¼ teaspoon ground nutmeg

2 cups whole-wheat bread cubes (from about 5 slices)

1 red apple, such as Fuji, peeled, cored, and chopped

1   Spray a 9-inch square baking dish with nonstick cooking spray.

2   In a large bowl, whisk together the milk, eggs, maple syrup, sugar, ginger, and nutmeg until well blended.

3   Stir in the bread cubes and apples. Pour the mixture into the baking dish, cover, and refrigerate for 1 hour.

4   Preheat the oven to 350°F.

5   Bake the pudding, uncovered, until the top browns and the custard sets, about 45 minutes. Serve warm.

SUBSTITUTION TIP: *Pears work well in place of apples in this recipe. If using pears, replace the maple syrup with honey and the nutmeg with cinnamon.*

PER SERVING Calories: 336; Total Fat: 4g; Saturated Fat: 1g; Sodium: 248mg; Carbohydrates: 64g; Fiber: 3g; Protein: 13g

Apple Crisp

PREP TIME: 15 MINUTES / COOK TIME: 1 HOUR

Apple crisp is a deeply satisfying dessert. With a fragrant spiced apple filling and a crunchy sweet oatmeal topping, it's the perfect dessert for fall when apples are at their peak of ripeness. Fuji apples are perfect for this recipe, because they maintain a tender crisp texture when cooked. Serves 8

Nonstick cooking spray

2 red apples, such as Fuji, peeled, cored, and chopped

1 teaspoon grated fresh ginger

½ teaspoon ground cinnamon

¼ teaspoon ground nutmeg

Pinch salt

1½ tablespoons unsalted butter, cut into small pieces

⅓ cup all-purpose flour

⅓ cup old-fashioned oats

⅓ cup brown sugar

1   Preheat the oven to 375°F.

2   Spray a 9-inch square baking dish with nonstick cooking spray.

3   In a medium bowl, toss the apples with the ginger, cinnamon, nutmeg, and salt until combined.

4   Spread the apples in the prepared baking dish.

5   In another bowl, mix the butter, flour, oats, and brown sugar. Use your hands to mix, pinching between your fingers to evenly distribute the butter.

6   Spread the mixture evenly over the top of the apples.

7   Bake until the topping is browned, about 1 hour. Serve warm.

SUBSTITUTION TIP: *Pears work well in place of apples in this recipe. The pears have a milder, slightly sweeter flavor than the apples.*

PER SERVING Calories: 112; Total Fat: 3g; Saturated Fat: 2g; Sodium: 37mg; Carbohydrates: 21g; Fiber: 2g; Protein: 2g

Orange Crème Brûlée

PREP TIME: 10 MINUTES, PLUS ABOUT 2 HOURS FOR COOLING AND CHILLING / COOK TIME: 40 MINUTES

Creamy crème brûlée, with its burnt-sugar shell, is a delicious dessert, but it is usually loaded with fat. This recipe uses nonfat Greek yogurt to lighten it up, while orange zest adds a subtle but delicious orange flavor. Serves 4

1 cup nonfat milk

¼ cup plain nonfat Greek yogurt

1 large egg

2 large egg whites

½ teaspoon alcohol-free vanilla

1 teaspoon grated orange zest

¼ cup sugar, plus 4 teaspoons more for sprinkling

1 Preheat the oven to 350°F.

2 Pour about 1 inch of boiling water into a 9-inch square baking dish and carefully put the baking dish in the oven to create a water bath.

3 In a medium bowl, whisk together all of the ingredients, except for 4 teaspoons of the sugar, until well combined.

4 Pour the mixture into four 5-ounce ramekins and carefully set the ramekins in the prepared water bath in the oven.

5 Bake until the custard is set in the middle but still slightly jiggly on the outside, about 40 minutes.

6 Carefully transfer the ramekins to a wire rack to cool for 30 minutes, then chill them in the refrigerator for at least 1 hour and as long as 24 hours.

7 Preheat the broiler. ▸

8   Sprinkle the tops of the chilled crème brûlées with the remaining 4 teaspoons of sugar.

9   Broil the crème brûlées just until the sugar hardens and begins to brown, about 4 minutes. Serve.

COOKING TIP: *Water baths help slow cooking for delicate dishes like custards. To keep the ramekins from slipping around on the bottom of the water bath, line the bottom of the pan with a washcloth before adding the water.*

PER SERVING Calories: 104; Total Fat: 1g; Saturated Fat: 0g; Sodium: 76mg; Carbohydrates: 17g; Fiber: 0g; Protein: 6g

Maple-Ginger Pudding

**PREP TIME: 5 MINUTES, PLUS 3 HOURS FOR CHILLING /
COOK TIME: 10 MINUTES**

Who needs instant pudding when it's so easy to make a low-fat, creamy pudding on your stovetop in less than 15 minutes? Homemade pudding has so much more flavor than the instant type, and you can easily tailor it to your specific tastes. Serves 8

2 cups nonfat milk

¼ cup pure maple syrup

¼ cup brown sugar

½ teaspoon alcohol-free vanilla

1 teaspoon ground ginger

Pinch salt

3 tablespoons cornstarch

3 tablespoons water

1   In a large saucepan, cook the milk, syrup, brown sugar, and vanilla over medium-high heat, stirring constantly, until it comes to a boil, about 3 minutes.

2   Reduce the heat to medium-low and continue cooking, stirring constantly, for 1 minute.

3   Remove from the heat and stir in the ginger and salt.

4   In a small bowl, whisk together the cornstarch and water until smooth. Add this slurry to the mixture.

5   Return the pudding to medium-low heat and cook, stirring constantly, until it boils, about 3 minutes more. Continue boiling and stirring for 1 minute.

6   Pour the pudding into a bowl or individual custard cups and chill for 3 hours. Serve.

SUBSTITUTION TIP: *For a more intense maple flavor, replace the vanilla with imitation maple flavoring.*

PER SERVING Calories: 78; Total Fat: 0g; Saturated Fat: 0g; Sodium: 55mg; Carbohydrates: 17g; Fiber: 0g; Protein: 2g

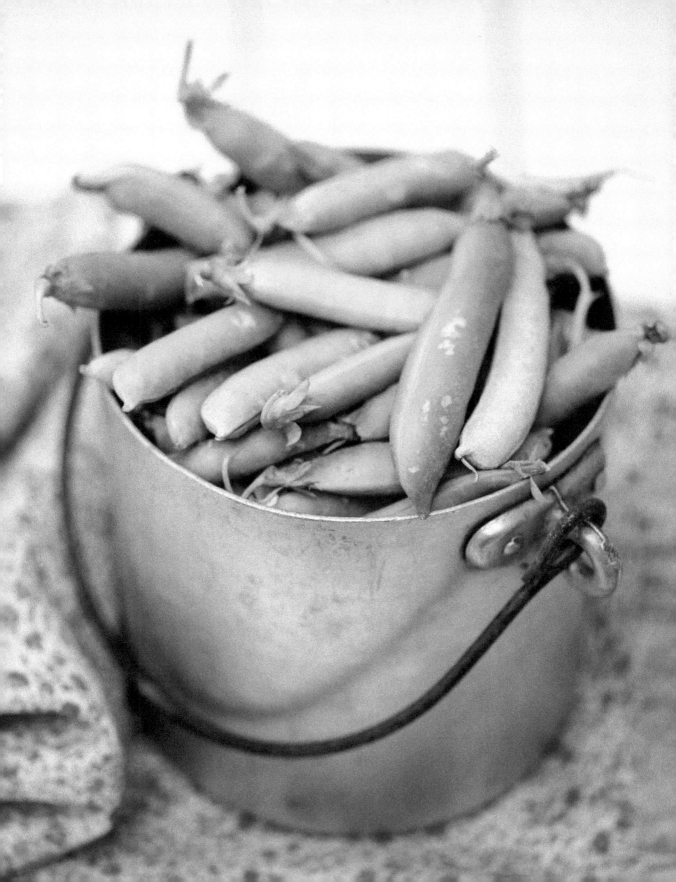

The FDA's Food pH List

Food	pH
Artichokes, fresh	5.6
Artichokes, canned	5.7 to 6.0
Asparagus, fresh	6.1 to 6.7
Asparagus, canned	5.2 to 5.3
Beans, green	4.6
Beans, lima	6.5
Beets, fresh	4.9 to 5.6
Beets, canned	4.9
Brussels sprouts	6.0 to 6.3
Cabbage, green	5.4 to 6.9
Cabbage, red	5.4 to 6.0
Cabbage, savoy	6.3
Cabbage, white	6.2
Carrots, fresh	4.9 to 5.2
Carrots, canned	5.2
Cauliflower	5.6
Celery	5.7 to 6.0
Corn, fresh	6.0 to 7.5
Corn, canned	6.0
Cucumbers	5.1 to 5.7
Cucumbers, pickled	3.2 to 3.5
Eggplant	4.5 to 5.3
Hominy	6.0

VEGETABLES

Food	pH
Kale	6.4 to 6.8
Kohlrabi	5.7 to 5.8
Leeks	5.5 to 6.0
Lettuce	5.8 to 6.0
Mushrooms	6.2
Okra	5.5 to 6.4
Olives, black	6.0 to 6.5
Olives, green	3.6 to 3.8
Onions, red	5.3 to 5.8
Onions, white	5.4 to 5.8
Onions, yellow	5.4 to 5.6
Parsnips	5.3
Peas, fresh	5.8 to 7.0
Peas, frozen	6.4 to 6.7
Peas, canned	5.7 to 6.0
Peppers, bell	5.2
Potatoes, russet	6.1
Potatoes, sweet	5.3 to 5.6
Pumpkin	4.8 to 5.2
Radishes, red	5.8 to 6.5
Radishes, white	5.5 to 5.7
Rhubarb	3.1 to 3.4
Sauerkraut	3.5 to 3.6

VEGETABLES

	Food	pH
VEGETABLES	Spinach, fresh	5.5 to 6.8
	Spinach, frozen	6.3 to 6.5
	Squash	5.5 to 6.0
	Tomatoes, fresh	4.2 to 4.9
	Tomatoes, canned	3.5 to 4.7
	Tomato juice	4.1 to 4.2
	Tomato paste	3.5 to 4.7
	Turnips	5.2 to 5.5
	Zucchini	5.8 to 6.1
HERBS	Chives	5.2 to 6.1
	Horseradish	5.3
	Parsley	5.7 to 6.0
	Sorrel	3.7
GRAINS AND LEGUMES	Beans, kidney	5.4 to 6.0
	Bread	5.3 to 5.8
	Cake	5.2 to 8.0
	Crackers	7.0 to 8.5
	Flour	6.0 to 6.3
	Lentils	6.3 to 6.8
	Rice, brown	6.2 to 6.7
	Rice, white	6.0 to 6.7
	Rice, wild	6.0 to 6.4
FRUITS	Apples	3.3 to 3.9
	Apple juice	3.4 to 4.0
	Applesauce	3.3 to 3.6
	Apricots, fresh	3.3 to 4.0
	Apricots, dried	3.6 to 4.0
	Apricots, canned	3.7
	Bananas	4.5 to 5.2
	Blackberries	3.2 to 4.5
	Blueberries, fresh	3.7
	Blueberries, frozen	3.1 to 3.4
	Cantaloupe	6.2 to 7.1
	Cherries	3.2 to 4.1
	Cranberry sauce	2.4

	Food	pH
FRUITS	Cranberry juice	2.3 to 2.5
	Dates	6.3 to 6.6
	Figs	4.6
	Grapefruit	3.0 to 3.3
	Grapes	3.4 to 4.5
	Lemons	2.2 to 2.4
	Limes	1.8 to 2.0
	Mango	3.9 to 4.6
	Melons, honeydew	6.3 to 6.7
	Nectarines	3.9
	Oranges	3.1 to 4.1
	Orange juice	3.6 to 4.3
	Papaya	5.2 to 5.7
	Peaches, fresh	3.4 to 3.6
	Peaches, jarred	4.2
	Peaches, canned	4.9
	Persimmons	5.4 to 5.8
	Pineapple, fresh	3.3 to 5.2
	Pineapple, canned	3.5
	Plums	2.8 to 4.6
	Pomegranates	3.0
	Prunes	3.1 to 5.4
	Prune juice	3.7
	Raspberries	3.2 to 3.7
	Strawberries, fresh	3.0 to 3.5
	Strawberries, frozen	2.3 to 3.0
	Tangerines	4.0
	Watermelon	5.2 to 5.8
DAIRY	Butter	6.1 to 6.4
	Buttermilk	4.5
	Milk	6.3 to 8.5
	Cream	6.5
	Cheese, camembert	7.4
	Cheese, cheddar	5.9
	Cheese, cottage	5.0

	Food	pH
DAIRY	Cheese, cream	4.9
	Cheese, Edam	5.4
	Cheese, Roquefort	5.5 to 5.9
	Cheese, Swiss	5.1 to 6.6
	Eggs, whites	7.0 to 9.0
	Eggs, yolks	6.4
	Eggs, whole	7.1 to 7.9
MEAT, POULTRY, FISH	Beef, ground	5.1 to 6.2
	Beef, steak	5.8 to 7.0
	Chicken	6.5 to 6.7
	Clams	6.5
	Crab	7.0
	Fish	6.6 to 7.3
	Ham	5.9 to 6.1
	Lamb	5.4 to 6.7
	Oysters	4.8 to 6.3
	Pork	5.3 to 6.9
	Salmon	6.1 to 6.3
	Shrimp	6.8 to 7.0
	Tuna	5.2 to 6.1
	Turkey	5.7 to 6.8
	Veal	6.0
	Whitefish	5.5

	Food	pH
OTHER	Cider	2.9 to 3.3
	Cocoa	6.3
	Corn syrup	5.0
	Cornstarch	4.0 to 7.0
	Ginger ale	2.0 to 4.0
	Honey	3.9
	Jam	3.1 to 3.5
	Mayonnaise	4.2 to 4.5
	Molasses	5.0 to 5.5
	Raisins	3.8 to 4.0
	Sugar	5.0 to 6.0
	Vinegar	2.0 to 3.5
	Yeast	3.0 to 3.5

What to Expect at the Doctor's Office

The first step in dealing with severe or chronic acid reflux is to visit your doctor. Typically, you will first see your primary care physician, who may refer you to an otolaryngologist (ear, nose, and throat doctor, or ENT) or a gastroenterologist, depending on how your symptoms affect you.

To prepare for your doctor's visit, keep a journal of foods you eat and symptoms they trigger so you can clearly demonstrate to your doctor exactly how your acid reflux functions. Remember to take lists of any medications, herbs, vitamins, and supplements you take so your doctor has a full health picture.

Tests

Your doctor will ask pertinent questions that may include information about foods you eat, frequency of flare-ups, specific symptoms, and any contributing factors such as stress, alcohol, or smoking. Your doctor will likely perform a brief examination.

Medication

If your primary care physician recognizes your symptoms as acid reflux, he or she may at first recommend some type of medication (either prescription or over the counter, such as an H_2 blocker or a PPI. Your doctor may also offer dietary and lifestyle suggestions to help you manage your symptoms.

When you get your medication from either the pharmacist or the drugstore, be sure to read all of the package insert information, which will tell you how much and when you should take the medication, as well as providing information about any side effects.

In some cases, your doctor may recommend further evaluation from a specialist such as a gastroenterologist or an ENT. Bring the same information to these specialists that you shared with your primary care physician, including any information about medications that were prescribed and how they have affected your symptoms.

The specialist may wish to perform additional tests.

Acid Monitoring

Known as an ambulatory acid probe test, your doctor may use a device to monitor the amount of acid in your esophagus for a 24-hour period as you go about your day. There are a few different types of probes used in this test, including a chip the doctor places in your throat during an endoscopy that transmits information about pH levels. If your doctor administers this test, you will also carry a small computer to receive the signals so your doctor can evaluate the pH levels. The chip used in this test passes through your alimentary canal and will pass in a bowel movement a few days after it was placed.

A less invasive way to monitor acid in the esophagus is by inserting a small, flexible catheter through one of your nostrils and into your esophagus. The doctor then attaches a small computer to the tube to receive signals about the amount of acid in your esophagus. After 24 hours, the doctor removes the tube and examines the results.

Both of these are outpatient procedures, and you return to normal life for the 24 hours that the computer monitors your pH.

X-Rays

Your doctor can also examine your upper digestive system with an X-ray. During this procedure, you will need to swallow liquid barium, which is thick and chalky. The liquid will coat your digestive tract so the X-rays can more easily visualize what is happening. This procedure usually takes about an hour, and you can return to your normal life when it ends.

Endoscopy

Your doctor may wish to gain a clearer picture by using an endoscope. An endoscope is a small, thin, flexible tube with a camera that is inserted through your mouth to look in your esophagus and upper digestive system.

During an endoscopy, you may receive an injection of sedating medicine, and your doctor may also spray your mouth with a local anesthesia. The tube may be inserted through a plastic mouth guard to keep you from biting down on it during the procedure. Your doctor will ask you to swallow the tube to help with insertion. While the procedure might provoke some anxiety, it typically doesn't cause any pain.

In order to help the doctor see better, he or she may puff some air into the esophagus to open it up. The doctor may also use tools to gather tissue samples. The procedure won't take much longer than 20 minutes, and in some cases it can be over in as few as 5 minutes.

Esophageal Manometry

This test allows your doctor to determine how well your esophagus works by measuring muscular contractions. During this test, the doctor passes a thin flexible tube through your nose into your esophagus in order to determine how well the muscle contracts and relaxes.

During the procedure, your doctor will spray anesthetic in your throat and/or nose. After inserting the tube, the doctor will ask you to swallow water in order to measure how well the esophagus works. The test takes about 30 minutes.

Treatments

After appropriate testing, your doctor will make a plan to manage your acid reflux. This plan may include medications like antacids, PPIs, or H_2 blockers.

Depending on the severity of your condition, your doctor may suggest over-the-counter medications, or he or she may prescribe prescription-strength drugs.

Your doctor may also recommend lifestyle and dietary changes, such as elevating the head of your bed and eliminating spicy foods as a way of managing your GERD.

Some cases of GERD may require surgical intervention. Surgical procedures strengthen or reinforce the LES. These are typically outpatient procedures performed under general anesthesia. The doctor uses a laparoscope in these minimally invasive procedures.

Whatever tests and treatments your doctor recommends, working in conjunction with health care professionals while managing diet and lifestyle can help you minimize or eliminate the symptoms of acid reflux.

Conversion Tables

VOLUME EQUIVALENTS (LIQUID)

U.S. Standard	US Standard (ounces)	Metric (approximate)
2 tablespoons	1 fl. oz.	30 mL
¼ cup	2 fl. oz.	60 mL
½ cup	4 fl. oz.	120 mL
1 cup	8 fl. oz.	240 mL
1½ cups	12 fl. oz.	355 mL
2 cups or 1 pint	16 fl. oz.	475 mL
4 cups or 1 quart	32 fl. oz.	1 L
1 gallon	128 fl. oz.	4 L

OVEN TEMPERATURES

Fahrenheit (F)	Celsius (C) (approximate)
250°	120°
300°	150°
325°	165°
350°	180°
375°	190°
400°	200°
425°	220°
450°	230°

VOLUME EQUIVALENTS (DRY)

U.S. Standard	Metric (approximate)
⅛ teaspoon	0.5 mL
¼ teaspoon	1 mL
½ teaspoon	2 mL
¾ teaspoon	4 mL
1 teaspoon	5 mL
1 tablespoon	15 mL
¼ cup	59 mL
⅓ cup	79 mL
½ cup	118 mL
⅔ cup	156 mL
¾ cup	177 mL
1 cup	235 mL
2 cups or 1 pint	475 mL
3 cups	700 mL
4 cups or 1 quart	1 L

WEIGHT EQUIVALENTS

U.S. Standard	Metric (approximate)
½ ounce	15 g
1 ounce	30 g
2 ounces	60 g
4 ounces	115 g
8 ounces	225 g
12 ounces	340 g
16 ounces or 1 pound	455 g

The Dirty Dozen and Clean Fifteen

A nonprofit environmental watchdog organization called Environmental Working Group (EWG) looks at data supplied by the U.S. Department of Agriculture (USDA) and the Food and Drug Administration (FDA) about pesticide residues. Each year it compiles a list of the best and worst pesticide loads found in commercial crops. You can use these lists to decide which fruits and vegetables to buy organic to minimize your exposure to pesticides and which produce is considered safe enough to buy conventionally. This does not mean they are pesticide-free, though, so wash these fruits and vegetables thoroughly.

These lists change every year, so make sure you look up the most recent one before you fill your shopping cart. You'll find the most recent lists as well as a guide to pesticides in produce at EWG.org/FoodNews.

2015 Dirty Dozen

Apples
Celery
Cherry tomatoes
Cucumbers
Grapes
Nectarines (imported)
Peaches
Potatoes
Snap peas (imported)
Spinach

Strawberries
Sweet bell peppers

In addition to the Dirty Dozen, the EWG added two types of produce contaminated with highly toxic organo-phosphate insecticides:
Kale/collard greens
Hot peppers

2015 Clean Fifteen

Asparagus
Avocados
Cabbage
Cantaloupes (domestic)
Cauliflower
Eggplants
Grapefruits
Kiwis
Mangoes
Onions

Papayas
Pineapples
Sweet corn
Sweet peas (frozen)
Sweet potatoes

References

Abbas, Abul K., Andrew H. Lichtman, and Shiv Pillai. *Basic Immunology: Functions and Disorders of the Immune System*. 4th ed. Philadelphia: Saunders, 2012.

American Academy of Otolaryngology–Head and Neck Surgery. "GERD and LPR." Accessed April 16, 2015. www.entnet.org/content/gerd-and-lpr.

American Autoimmune Related Diseases Association. "Autoimmune Statistics." Accessed April 15, 2015. www.aarda.org/autoimmune-information/autoimmune-statistics/.

Cleveland Clinic. "24-Hour Esophageal pH Test." Accessed April 17, 2015. http://my.clevelandclinic.org/health/diagnostics/hic_24-Hour_Esophageal_pH_Test.

Cleveland Clinic. "GERD or Acid Reflux or Heartburn Overview." Accessed April 16, 2015. http://my.clevelandclinic.org/health/diseases_conditions/hic_gastroesophogeal_reflux_disease_GERD/dd_overview.

DiMarino, Michael C. Florida Hospital. "Statistics about Heartburn." Accessed April 16, 2015 www.floridahospital.com/heartburn-gerd/statistics.

Gaude, Gajanan S. "Pulmonary Manifestations of Gastroesophageal Reflux Disease." *Annals of Thoracic Medicine* 4, no. 3 (July 2009): 115–23. doi: 10.4103/1817-1737.53347.

Halmos, E. P., V. A. Power, S. J. Shepherd, P. R. Gibson, and J. G. Muir. "A Diet Low in FODMAPs Reduces Symptoms of Irritable Bowel Syndrome." *Gastroenterology* (January 2014). doi: 10.1053/j.gastro.2013.09.046.

Heidelbaugh, Joel J., Andrea H. Kim, Robert Chang, and Paul C. Walker. "Overutilization of Proton-Pump Inhibitors: What the Clinician Needs to Know." *Therapeutic Advances in Gastroenterology* 5, no. 4 (July 2012): 219–32. doi: 10.1177/1756283X12437358.

International Foundation for Functional Gastrointestinal Disorders. "Laryngeal Pharyngeal Reflux (LPR)." Accessed April 15, 2015. www.aboutgerd.org/site/symptoms/lpr.

Kemps, E., M. Tiggerman, and S. Bettany. "Non-Food Odorants Reduce Chocolate Cravings." *Appetite* 58, no. 3 (June 2012): 1087–90. doi: 10.1016/j.appet.2012.03.002.

Koufman, Jamie and Jordan Stern. *Dropping Acid: The Reflux Diet Cookbook & Cure*. New York: Katalitix Publishing, 2010.

The Low-FODMAP 28-Day Plan. Berkeley, CA: Rockridge Press, 2014.

Mayo Clinic. "GERD: Symptoms." Accessed April 16, 2015. www.mayoclinic.org /diseases-conditions/gerd/basics /symptoms/con-20025201.

Mayo Clinic. "GERD: Treatments and Drugs." Accessed April 16, 2015. www .mayoclinic.org/diseases-conditions /gerd/basics/treatment/con-20025201.

Mayo Clinic. "Histamine H_2 Antagonist (Oral Intravenous Route)." Accessed April 14, 2015. www.mayoclinic.org/drugs -supplements/histamine-h2-antagonist -oral-route-injection-route -intravenous-route/side-effects /drg-20068584

Mayo Clinic. "Upper Endoscopy: What You Can Expect." Accessed April 17, 2015. www.mayoclinic.org/tests-procedures /endoscopy/basics/what-you-can -expect/PRC-20020363.

McKinley Health Center. "The GERD Diet (Gastroesophageal Reflux Disease)." Accessed April 16, 2015. www.mckinley .illinois.edu/handouts/gerd_diet.html.

MedlinePlus (U.S. National Library of Medicine). "Baclofen Oral." Accessed April 16, 2015. www.nlm.nih.gov/medlineplus /druginfo/meds/a682530.html.

MedlinePlus (U.S. National Library of Medicine). "H_2 Blockers." Accessed April 16, 2015. www.nlm.nih.gov /medlineplus/ency/patientinstructions /000382.htm.

MedlinePlus (U.S. National Library of Medicine). "Proton Pump Inhibitors." Accessed April 16, 2015. www.nlm .nih.gov/medlineplus/ency /patientinstructions/000381.htm.

MedlinePlus (U.S. National Library of Medicine). "Taking Antacids." Accessed April 16, 2015. www .nlm.nih.gov/medlineplus/ency /patientinstructions/000198.htm.

Merck Manual: Professional Version. "Overview of Acid Secretion." Accessed April 14, 2015. www.merckmanuals.com /professional/gastrointestinal-disorders /gastritis-and-peptic-ulcer-disease /overview-of-acid-secretion.

Nailboff, Brian D., M. Mayer, L. Z. Fitzgerald, L. Chang, R. Bolus, and E. A. Mayer. "The Effect of Life Stress on Symptoms of Heartburn." *Psychosomatic Medicine* 66, no. 3 (May 2004): 426–34. Accessed April 16, 2015. www.ncbi.nlm.nih.gov /pubmed/15184707.

National Institute of Diabetes and Digestive and Kidney Diseases. "Definition and Facts for Gastroesophageal Reflux (GER) and Gastroesophageal Reflux Disease (GERD)." Accessed April 16, 2015. www .niddk.nih.gov/health-information /health-topics/digestive-diseases /ger-and-gerd-in-adults/Pages /definition-facts.aspx.

National Institute of Diabetes and Digestive and Kidney Diseases. "Symptoms and Causes of Gastroesophageal Reflux (GER) and Gastroesophageal Reflux Disease (GERD)." Accessed April 16, 2015. www .niddk.nih.gov/health-information/ health-topics/digestive-diseases /ger-and-gerd-in-adults/Pages /symptoms-causes.aspx.

Norwegian University of Science and Technology. "Prevalence of Acid Reflux Has Increased by Half over the Past Decade." Accessed April 16, 2014. www .ntnu.edu/aboutntnu/ntnu-news-2012 /acid-reflux.

PDRhealth (Physicians' Desk Reference). "Gastroesophageal Reflux Disease (GERD) Symptoms." Accessed April 16, 2015. www.pdrhealth.com/diseases /gastroesophageal-reflux-disease-gerd /symptoms.

Robillard, Norman. *Fast Tract Digestion: Heartburn.* Watertown, MA: Self Health, 2012.

Tidwell, D. Wayne. "Reflux Symptom Index." Baylor Institute for Rehabilitation: Voice, Speech, and Swallowing Center.

U.S. Food and Drug Administration. "pH Values of Various Foods." Accessed April 16, 2015. www.fda.gov/Food /FoodborneIllnessContaminants /CausesOfIllnessBadBugBook /ucm122561.htm.

Wangen, Stephen. "A Hidden Epidemic: Reflux and Food Allergies." *Reflux Digest* 13, no. 2 (September 2009): 1, 10.

Yarandi, Shadi Sadeghi. "Overlapping Gastroesophageal Reflux Disease and Irritable Bowel Syndrome: Increased Dysfunctional Symptoms." *World Journal of Gastroenterology* 16, no. 10 (March 2010): 1232–38. doi: 10.3748/wjg .v16.i9.1232.

Index

About the Author

KAREN FRAZIER is a Seattle-based writer and nutrition and fitness expert who specializes in cookbooks for restrictive diets. Before being diagnosed with celiac disease and an acute dairy allergy, Karen suffered from severe gastro-intestinal symptoms, chronic GERD, malnutrition, and anemia for nearly two decades. It wasn't until she changed her diet that she finally found relief from her symptoms and improved her health. Karen is the author of several cookbooks, including *The Hashimoto's Cookbook and Action Plan* and *The Gastroparesis Cookbook*.

CPSIA information can be obtained
at www.ICGtesting.com
Printed in the USA
LVHW020424171220
674317LV00002B/5